Senior Fitness

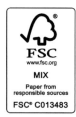

FSC

www.fsc.org

MIX

Paper from
responsible sources

FSC® C013483

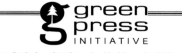

green
press
INITIATIVE

Senior Fitness

The Diet and Exercise Program
for Maximum Health and Longevity

Ruth E. Heidrich, PhD

Lantern Books · New York
A Division of Booklight Inc.

2005
Lantern Books
One Union Square West, Suite 201
New York, NY 10003

Copyright Ruth Heidrich, 2005

This book is not intended to diagnose, prescribe or treat any medical conditions. Always consult your health care provider before initiating any health or fitness program.

Cover photo: Running at Macchu Picchu. Photograph by Bob Leitch.
Cover design by Josh Hooten.

Printed in the United States of America

Library of Congress Cataloging-in-Publication Data
Heidrich, Ruth E.
Senior fitness : the diet and exercise program for maximum health and longevity / by Ruth E. Heidrich.—1st ed.
p. cm.
Includes bibliographical references.
ISBN 1-59056-074-4 (alk. paper)
1. Older people—Health and hygiene. 2. Physical fitness for older people. 3. Exercise for older people. I. Title.
RA777.6.H46 2005
613.7'1'0846—dc22
2004025931

TABLE OF CONTENTS

❧

INTRODUCTION

ON JULY 5, 1982, at the age of forty-seven, I got the shock of my life: I was told I had breast cancer. As a woman who considered herself a health-conscious eater and had run marathons, I thought I couldn't possibly get sick—let alone get cancer! I considered myself to be extremely healthy and certainly was the fittest person I knew. But health is like oxygen in that you tend not to notice it until it's no longer there. Now it seemed all the air had suddenly been sucked out of the room, and I was gasping for breath.

I was undergoing a biopsy to remove a lump in my breast, which I was sure would be benign; I'd had several mammograms, and they had all come out negative. (Besides, it was easier to think that things like cancer happened to *other* people.) I insisted on no general anesthesia because I wanted to be awake to know and see exactly what was going on. I watched the surgeon make the first incision. Then, going deeper and deeper, he finally reached the tumor, cut a wide margin around it, and pulled out the whole bloody mass. The gruesome sight embedded itself indelibly in my brain. I watched, unable to take my eyes off that "thing" that had been growing in my breast, as the surgeon, scalpel in hand, cut the tumor in half to see what the inside looked like.

When he uttered an ominous "Uh-oh," I was gripped by panic and almost leaped off the operating table. "What do you mean, 'uh-oh'?" I said. As he realized that he'd forgotten this particular patient was awake, the doctor explained that what he had seen did not look good. The tumor was the size of a golf ball and appeared full of what looked like grains of sand. The grains of "sand," he said, were calcifications—cancer cells that my body had tried to wall off and encapsulate.

I had breast cancer. I turned cold and numb with fear. It was like an immediate death sentence. In my fright, I was trying desperately to think logically. All I wanted to do initially was to turn control over to my surgeon, thinking that my life was in his hands. I remember hearing the words come out of my mouth, "What do we do now?"

It was only after the surgery, when the doctor turned me over to an oncologist (a specialist in cancer), that I realized my surgeon really didn't know that much about breast cancer treatment. He wasn't even supposed to; it was not his area of expertise. His specialty was surgery (amputating breasts, actually), not treating cancer. The oncologist, however, was not much more help. When I asked him why I had gotten cancer when I was taking such good care of myself, he said, "We don't know." When I asked what I could do to strengthen my immune system to fight the cancer, again he said, "We just don't know."

And it wasn't just him. I sought a second, third, fourth, and even a fifth opinion and got the same answer: "We don't know." My prognosis varied, depending on whom I talked to, but all agreed that this was an aggressive, life-threatening cancer, and my chance of survival depended on how far it had spread. Because there were no clear margins, meaning that the cancer had spread beyond what the surgeon had removed, more surgery was required. After I had the second surgery, a modified radical mastectomy, the surgeon said that he thought he'd gotten all the cancer in my breast since there was no breast tissue left. However, no one could say at that point whether it had spread *beyond* the breast until they completed scans for the bone, liver, lung, and brain—the most common places for its fatal spread.

MOTIVATION

Seeing the cancer literally right in front of me was not only a huge shock but also provided me with a very strong motivator. I did *not* want to die. I resolved to do everything in my power to fight this disease.

At that point in my life, my career was taking off: I was a GS-13 government worker who had just been chosen for a program that was to prepare me for the top echelons of our government. I thought I was taking good care of myself, knowing I had good genes. After all, all four of my grandparents lived into their nineties. I thought that genes were all-important and that I would live as long as they had despite the fact that they had heart disease, cancer, arthritis, Type 2 diabetes, and osteoporosis. Of course, I wasn't going to make my genes do all the work; I'd become a daily runner, knowing that getting some exercise was important. I'd given up red meat, switching to chicken and fish to get what I was told was lots of "high-quality" protein. I drank skim milk "for my bones," did monthly breast self exams—all the things I'd read were important to maintaining good health.

What was not average about me was that I was a voracious reader, particularly of things like medical journals. I'd studied hard, earned a master's degree in psychology and was on my way to my doctorate, which required that I take courses in statistics, research design, and experimental techniques. They were difficult for me and I hated them, but I never dreamed that they would one day save my life, as they enabled me to learn what I needed to know to regain my health.

In fact, I was about to learn a valuable lesson: that I alone was responsible for my own health care. No more just blindly following platitudes such as "Get your mammograms," because mammograms sure missed this one. As I discovered, you cannot just turn all responsibility over to doctors and the medical system.

After I had visited the doctors, I read about Dr. John McDougall and his research into the effects of diet on breast cancer. I immediately went to see him. Dr. McDougall said that any tumor of a size large enough to be clinically detectable had probably been there long enough to have been shedding cancerous cells for six to eight or even ten years. Discouraged, I began to fear that there was absolutely no hope. Dr. McDougall then told me that if I wanted to save my life, I had to change my diet. I was positive that it was too late, since I must have had this cancer for several years by that time, but he repeated the words, "If you want to save your life, change your diet." I enrolled in the clinical research study that he was conducting and started a vegan (no animal products), low-fat diet that day.

I refused chemotherapy and radiation because McDougall's clinical study required no other variable than the dietary change and my oncologist could not provide any evidence that either chemotherapy or radiation would make a difference in my prognosis and length of survival. However, I was definitely not content to just sit back and wait to see if the cancer had spread to my bones, lungs, liver, and brain—as it later turned out, it had, since I had positive scans, meaning there were signs of cancer in my bones and one lung. I set about trying to learn all I could about the disease, talking to anybody who I thought might have some answers, making long-distance calls all over the country and spending hours in the medical library. In a newspaper page full of fine print, the words "breast cancer" would jump out at me. I had become obsessed with the disease. It was all I could think about, night and day.

What I learned was riveting. I became 100 percent convinced that this disease that now strikes one out of eight American women[1] is related to our diet. As I made what I thought then were radical changes in my diet, I was astonished to feel that, as if for the first time, my body was being properly fueled. The proof of this was in my running times. Although I was getting older, I was getting faster!

Then I started getting angry. Why had I had to discover this myself? I had had to dig out most of the information on my own, using my graduate school training, without which I could never have plowed through all that data in the professional journals. Doctors like John McDougall were few and far between, and, besides, my oncologist (and everybody else, including husband, relatives, and friends) disparaged everything that I'd been told by Dr. McDougall.

It still makes me angry to think of all those other women who were told nothing about their disease and what caused it. When I ask other breast cancer patients what type of breast cancer they have, they invariably say, "I didn't even know there *were* different kinds of breast cancer." Why aren't these women being told that if they hadn't been eating the Standard American Diet (ironically called "SAD," or "the SAD diet"), they probably would not have gotten cancer? When they are offered options for treatment after surgery, it is usually only chemotherapy and radiation. Why aren't they told they are risking permanent damage to their immune system and that there's no evidence that it will extend their lives?[2] Why aren't they being told that their best chance to save their lives is to change their diet?[3] An even greater irony is that of the few doctors who do know this, most of them are unwilling to spend the time required to explain to their patients the importance of diet. They assume that few of their patients will give up the rich foods that gave them their disease in the first place.

I wondered why this information wasn't on the front pages of every newspaper in the country. Why aren't people being told that what they're eating is *killing* them? How come there isn't an "operations manual" that tells us how this wonderful body of ours works? How do we do the "preventive maintenance" that will enable our body to go for 200,000 miles without blowing its engine? How do we keep the fuel lines from getting clogged up? Why is it that most people don't even know the proper kind of fuel to put in the body's gas tank?

GETTING FIT

The diet was my first response to cancer. The second was to complete my first Ironman Triathlon two years after my diagnosis. Now I have been cancer-free for twenty-two years. And that's not all. In 1998, at the age of sixty-three, I was named one of the Top Ten Fittest Women in North America by *Living Fit* magazine (the other nine were all under thirty-five years of age). At five-foot-eight inches tall and 125 pounds, I have a Body Mass Index (BMI) of nineteen, which is generally considered the ideal range for body composition. My blood pressure averages 90/60, which means that my arteries are very elastic and essentially wide open for the blood to course through. My VO2max, which is the measure of my body's ability to process oxygen, is sixty-six, one of the highest ever measured at the Tripler Army General Hospital in Honolulu, Hawaii, where I live. My resting heart rate of forty-four beats per minute means that my heart beats very efficiently. My bone density greatly exceeds that of a thirty-year-old female at peak bone density. My risk of heart attack, stroke, diabetes, hypertension (or high blood pressure), and hip fracture is extremely low. And nearly all of this is, I believe, due to my very healthy diet and an enjoyable daily exercise routine. That diet and exercise regimen is the heart of this book.

My aim in the previous paragraph is not to boast, but to show you how far I've come and to give you an insight into the central message of this book: that good health can be yours no matter what your previous medical history or how old you are. That might seem a remarkable statement to make and, quite rightly, you may be skeptical. After all, we're bombarded on a daily basis on television and radio, in the print media, and on the street with promises of miracle cures effected by one product or another. That skepticism is a good thing. In the next few paragraphs I'm going to try to answer the questions that are probably buzzing through your mind.

You might be saying to yourself, "Well, she has admitted that her grandparents lived into their nineties, so perhaps that's why she's alive." I can assure you, my *cancer* genes are no better than anyone else's. My fitness levels and my current cancer-free status are not the result of genetic "abnormality" but of the application of the principles I've learned over many years about the healthiest possible lifestyle. You should know that I made some mistakes along the way. However, I learned something from every one of them, and I feel much healthier and wiser as a result.

Second, I am *not* offering any miracle cures or peddling any drugs. You won't need to spend any more money or do anything outlandish or dangerous. What I can promise is that, if you follow my diet and fitness recommendations, you will lower your risk of disease.

Third, you should also know that I have had setbacks in my recovery from my double mastectomy and throughout the last two decades. Early on, I found out that the cancer in my breast had spread and that because my cholesterol level was so high I was at risk for a heart attack as well. Because of the diet I adopted, my cholesterol level fell to a level low enough that I am virtually immune to heart attacks. Consequently, I'm still here, life has never been better, and I've never been healthier.

Fourth, you may be wondering what qualifications I have to write this book. I'm not an MD and I'm not a professional nutritionist; my PhD is in health education. My response to that question is twofold.

First of all, I have *lived* my experiment—I have studied myself (and have been studied by doctors) for decades. I know *firsthand* how important it is to get full and accurate information about your health, and I also know that some members of the medical profession don't know what you need to know to maintain optimal health and wellness. That's why I did a lot of my own research—poring over the medical textbooks and journals so you don't have to.

Not only have I been doing all this myself for more than twenty years, but I've persuaded other folks to change their lives, and they've raved about how well the program works, even inviting me to speak to groups that they belong to, so we can share this information with them.

My conclusion is straightforward: Based on all my own research and the research of others, I feel confident in saying that attaining true fitness and empowering the latter half of our lives *both mentally and physically* is impossible without the foundation of a healthy, disease-free body.

UNHEALTHY HABITS

The last sentence of the previous paragraph may seem an unremarkable statement until you understand that an older, healthy, disease-free body is almost impossible to find in this country. Our lifestyle is riddled with unhealthy habits, most of which are actually *promoted* by our government, medical system, the pharmaceutical industry, and, unwittingly, by us. Take what we eat, for instance. We are given the wrong information about diet due to several critical factors. First, the meat, dairy, soft drink, and processed food industries have a major influence in determining government policy toward food. Second, the medical system is becoming more and more concerned with being a profitable business than with public health. Third, pharmaceutical companies wield unbelievable power over the health-care system. And, fourth, we *for the most part* think that the food, medical and drug industries all have the noble goal of "helping" us!

I know these are strong statements, but as you read this book you will see that what I say is hard to deny. You can only lay the foundation for a healthy maturity if you have the information that tells you how to do it. This is my second response to the question of why I am qualified to write this book. I'm not only going to talk about the importance of owning a healthy, disease-free body; I'm also going to emphasize how necessary it is for you to develop critical thinking, a skill we seem to have lost in this society.

Critical thinking means identifying the problem, looking at different possible causes of that problem, seeing possible solutions, examining and testing the evidence "for" and "against" those solutions, and, while trying to eliminate all bias, picking the solution and applying it objectively. This is much harder to do than most people think, because we *all* have unrecognized biases and unquestioned assumptions. A good example of an unquestioned assumption that many people hold is that meat is necessary in a healthful diet. Yet there's much scientific evidence to show that meat not only is not necessary but can actually be harmful. You will see some of this evidence throughout the book.

As you practice critical thinking, you may find many other examples to apply in your own thinking and in others' as well. Learn to question authority and don't be taken in by advertising. You should also question assumptions—your own and everybody else's. Critical thinking is a skill that will serve you very well for the rest of your life. I invite you to practice this skill as you read this book. In fact, I don't want you to just *read* it; I want you to underline crucial passages, highlight things to remember, and keep it by your bedside for frequent review and, I hope, inspiration. Don't take what I say for granted, either; visit the sources I cite and examine the data.

You can talk to plastic surgeons, exercise physiologists, beauty experts, nutritionists, medical doctors, and others about health and physical wellness, but I believe my approach is safer and more effective, and will save you money. Is this an exaggerated promise? Hype? A sales pitch? No, I don't think so. What I've done is to pull together information from many different sources with an eye to scientific credibility and put it together into a plan that you will find very easy to follow. Much of the information I present here may already be available, but it is scattered in medical journals, unpublished research, and on dusty library shelves. I have tried to be as scientific as possible in assessing the accuracy of the information presented here, as the last thing I want to do is to pass on any myths or misinformation. In any case, I invite the reader to view the data with an open mind, take what applies, and leave the rest, maybe, for later.

YOUR RACE FOR LIFE

You may not know it yet, but you *are* in a race for life, and it started the day you were born. As ill prepared as you were, you toed up to the starting line. Ready or not, the starter's gun fired, and off you ran.

If you had looked at the competitors around you, you would have seen a large crowd. Besides lots of other people, running behind and beside you were heart disease, strokes, all different kinds of cancer, diabetes, arthritis, osteoporosis, infections, accidents, obesity, aging—competitors that could keep you from making it to the finish line of life, or (almost as bad) affect the quality of your race. Any of the above will slow you down and keep you from having your best possible race. They can cause you agonizing pain and make your race miserable; or, worst of all, they can make you stumble and fall and drop out of the race, so that you never get the opportunity to express the potential that you have lying within you.

Let me emphasize the following: *What you'll find in the following chapters has the power to transform your life.* You will find the secret to having a slim, attractive, strong body no matter how old you are. You will discover the secret to being able to eat as much as you want, never having to deny your natural, healthy appetite for food. Your energy levels will soar and yet you'll need less sleep, because you'll be getting a slumber that is deeper and of higher quality. You will learn the secrets to avoiding all those "competitors" listed above who may be sticking out a foot to trip you or your friends and relatives.

Once you learn and apply all this, you'll realize that you've never been so healthy in your life, and you'll wonder—and maybe even get really angry about—why no one ever told you these things before. I'm talking to you as someone who's been there— one who's had to become an expert in the fields of nutrition, exercise, and the psychology that makes us do what we do. It troubles me more than I can say that people are killing themselves just as their race for life gets started or stumbling and falling long before the halfway point. I want to be one of their coaches, telling them what pitfalls to avoid and cheering them on, even pulling them along if need be. After reading this book, maybe you will be a coach, too.

Until then, since you probably don't have your own personal coach, let me be yours. Don't wait another day to make a change, because the exciting changes I promise will happen to your body will start to happen within hours. Literally, within *hours*, your body will start to function like it's never functioned before— you'll feel more energetic, your blood will be thinner, and, for starters, you will probably suffer less from indigestion, heartburn, and constipation. Like me, you'll get mad and ask, "How come nobody ever told me this before?"

You should know also that it's never too late to start. No matter how badly you may have abused that poor body of yours, it is quite forgiving. Do you notice that no matter how many times you cut yourself, your body doesn't complain but starts immediately to work, healing each cut? Well, you've accumulated a lifetime of "cuts," and your poor body has been trying desperately to keep up with the self-inflicted injuries. If you've been living the standard American lifestyle, you may as well have been eating broken glass for all the cuts you've inflicted.

So resolve to stop the injuries to your body right this minute. What I will tell you in this book is what to eat instead of "broken glass"—how to help your body heal your "cuts." Not only will you stop and reverse the disease process but, even more, you will learn how to train your body so that it will maximize its performance. You'll even learn the strategies of "racing," so that if you do everything you read in here, you're going to be the champion in your race for life.

Each chapter in this book will cover a different affliction and show how both poor diet (disease) and lack of exercise (disuse) affect us and what we can do about it. Although all the research is not yet in, it is clear that nearly all chronic disease is preventable and reversible. Human bodies *are not meant to get sick or obese* and usually don't unless they're mistreated in some way. It is also very clear that the human body should not just wear out. Quite the opposite: The more the body gets "used," the longer it lasts. It's the *lack* of use that causes us to "rust out" and "crash." There will be some repetition between chapters because I want each chapter to be able to stand alone and there is so much interconnectedness between fitness, diet, exercise, and most diseases. In many instances, I will also be adding some of my own experiences as an illustration of how I know what I know.

It really is that easy. Come with me: I'll hold your hand; I'll cheer you on; you and I will do whatever it takes for you to have this wonderful, fully functioning body and the clear head to dream up goals that you never thought possible. Now, I'm *not* saying that you have to do the Ironman Triathlon, although please know that most of you could if you wanted to. What I *am* saying is that it's so easy to do a *lot* more than you're doing right now.

If your exercise is now limited to changing the TV channels with your remote, bending your elbow at the dining table, jumping to conclusions, and stretching the truth, you can start by walking around the block first thing every morning, after lunch, or before bed. I'm going to try to convince you to take the lid off your ambitions. Start visualizing yourself in this super-fit, lean, strong, energetic body that is capable of incredible athletic feats. If your diet consists of 100 percent junk food, let me mentally go with you on a shopping trip to get good, healthy foods available to eat any time you feel like it, and to eat as much as you want.

.   .   .

As I approach my seventieth year, with no decrease in my energy level or zest for life, it has become obvious to me that the consequences of aging—with or without a serious medical condition like cancer—do not have to involve the debilitating conditions that too often affect older people. Indeed, we can stop or even reverse those ailments that are traditionally put down to getting older. In twenty-two years of an extraordinary medical journey, I have learned that anyone can do what I've done, and it's my job to convince you that you, too, could also be one of the fittest, healthiest people around. Don't let your health be like the oxygen mentioned at the beginning of this chapter; take care of it before it's gone, and read on.

CHAPTER 1

WHAT IS SENIOR FITNESS?

IN HAWAII, WHERE I live, we have a lot of tourists. The other day I was out for my daily run and a car rolled up, the window rolled down, and a voice said, "Excuse me, can you tell me how to get to Waikiki Beach?" They were actually only a block away from the beach, but because they were unfamiliar with the territory, they were lost—very close, but still lost.

I have a simple question that I want you to ask yourself throughout this book: Are you a native or are you a tourist? For forty-seven years I was a tourist where cancer was concerned. Oh, I knew it was out there somewhere. However, the day I heard the surgeon repeating over the phone to the pathologist, "infiltrating ductal carcinoma," with that damning diagnosis, I was immediately transformed from a tourist to a native. Suddenly, I felt a whole lot different. More than twenty years later, I'm still a native where cancer is concerned, because you can never go back to being a tourist.

The day I found out I had breast cancer was the day I started to gain a vision, mission, and passion. Now, when I look at the world I see four out of five people who will succeed in killing themselves slowly—and some *not* so slowly. I see women giving themselves breast cancer, osteoporosis, and arthritis; I see men giving themselves heart attacks, prostate cancer and impotence; I see kids giving themselves diabetes, acne, and obesity. I see folks unable to move, creaking slowly into a state of frozen joints, knee and hip replacements, and permanent disability.

What I know is that it doesn't have to be that way. I can see with X-ray vision, right through to their bony skeleton, their muscles laid over and attaching to the bones—and the layers of fat. I know they could all be vibrantly healthy if they would only change their food choices and start exercising. I can see all that with the vision of a native.

Then there's the mission. I didn't hesitate one moment, nor would you, to tell that tourist that Waikiki Beach is one block straight ahead and turn right, because if you're a native you know all this and don't mind sharing it. Here's a story to tell you what I mean.

I was flying from Dallas, where I'd attended a conference, home to Honolulu. The trip consisted of three legs—Dallas to Albuquerque, Albuquerque to Los Angeles, and Los Angeles to Honolulu. I had a briefcase full of work—a lot of reading from all the material I'd picked up at the conference. I was feeling very satisfied because I'd sold all but two copies of my first book, *A Race for Life*, and I never want to let go of the last copy because wherever I go I always seem to need it to show someone the statistics on how chicken and fish are just as high in cholesterol as beef and pork.

As the plane reached its cruising altitude, I settled back into my seat. I couldn't help but overhear the two women next to me as they started chatting. The subject got around to bifocals and how they both had just started to wear them, and how they hated them—especially when they had to take them on and off to see close up and then far away, or even worse, to peer over them.

Bifocals are a dead giveaway to aging, and I knew exactly what they were talking about because I'd gone through the same thing a few years before.

I tried, believe me, to ignore my "mission" and not tell them my secret about how they could avoid bifocals, but it was no good. I not only had to tell them how they could avoid bifocals through monovision or laser surgery, but I also had to tell them how to avoid breast cancer, ovarian cancer, colon cancer, heart attacks, strokes, diabetes, arthritis, osteoporosis, and, since they were of that uncertain bifocal age, "power surges" (hot flashes) as well. There went my last two books.

I was consoling myself with the prospect of doing work on the two remaining legs of my flight when, on the next plane, the flight attendant asked my neighbor, a Korean lady, what she wanted to drink. When she replied that she wanted milk, I honestly could not let that one go, either. I knew that most Asians have a terrible time with dairy products, lacking the enzyme, lactase, needed to digest lactose in milk. I had to tell her about the association of milk with such problems as gastrointestinal bleeding, osteoporosis, arthritis, ovarian cancer, heart disease, and other illnesses. And here I was, completely out of books. Imagine my surprise when by the end of the flight and the "lecture," the woman reached into her purse, pulled out some bills, and asked me to mail her a book.

Well, at least there was one more leg to go. Surely I would be able to get some work done on the four-and-a-half hour flight to Honolulu. Walking down the aisle of the plane, I spied my seat and noted my next seatmate was another woman. She was a very attractive African-American woman, whom I estimated to weigh well over 200 pounds. Sure enough, by the time we had gotten to Honolulu, this lady had promised to give up all animal products and to start stationary cycling and running in water every day. The best news is that she wants us both to go on the Oprah Winfrey Show to show her "before" and "after" pictures, and start helping others.

As this woman changed from being a tourist to being a native, we moved together through a vision, mission and passion. My vision was of a 200-pound woman as a 130-pound woman. My mission is that that we're going to go nationwide and show people how they can do it, too. I also saw her passion—I sensed her mounting excitement and resolve. For most "tourists," the unknown seems very challenging, if not impossible. Establishing a new habit takes about twenty-one days, and once that routine of eating only plant foods and getting daily exercise gets established, people wonder in retrospect why it seemed so difficult for them. They then go on to tell others—they get the vision, mission, and passion and are no longer tourists.

As we touched down in Honolulu, I realized how easy it was to touch people's lives and how important it was to show them the way—after all, it's only one block and turn right to avoid heart disease, cancer, stroke, and diabetes. I also saw, on the positive side, how it is possible to increase people's self-esteem through nice, lean, beautiful bodies with abundant vital energy, and how they, too, then have the vision, the mission, and the passion.

Now you, my friend, can never go back to being a tourist— knowing all this makes you a native!

GETTING FIT

Many, if not most, people think that aging is inevitable and that it should be "accepted with grace." Others resort to plastic surgery for face-lifts, breast implants, and liposuction. They try risky treatments such as injections of Human Growth Hormone to stop the aging process and Botox (botulinum toxin) to decrease wrinkles. Or they may try to fight aging with simple denial (remember Jack Benny, who was perpetually thirty-nine?)! Billions of dollars are spent each year on potions, anti-wrinkle creams, weight-loss pills, supplements, and a myriad of products that promise to reverse the aging process. While some of these strategies may help for a while, based on the evidence I believe that the best approach is the one presented in this book.

Besides just the cosmetic approaches to dealing with aging, the ravages of the most common degenerative diseases that we face shorten and handicap our lives way before our bodies' natural decline. In addition, the cost of these degenerative diseases threatens to bankrupt our health-care system and possibly even our economy. Most of these problems, both cosmetic and medical, are related to our lifestyle practices and can be reversed.

IGNORANCE ISN'T BLISS

When asked what the number one cause of death in the United States is, most people answer "heart disease." In my opinion, the number one cause of death is *ignorance*. Because you're not allowed to put "ignorance" on a death certificate, however, a secondary cause such as heart attack or cancer is listed instead. Too many people waste their time and money on pills and potions and still don't get the results they seek because they are looking in the wrong places. We are bombarded by advertisements trying to separate us from our money, and we fall for the promises because most people don't have the scientific background or do the critical thinking required to sort out promise from reality. If people really had all the information they needed, they would not be dying from ignorance.

Everywhere we look, we see pills that offer relief from symptoms of an unhealthy lifestyle. Just walk down the aisle of any drug store or pharmacy and take note of the amazing array of antidotes for problems ranging from allergies to zits—and everything in between. Whether you have a headache, an overly acidic stomach, heartburn, nasal congestion, joint pain, insomnia, constipation, or hemorrhoids, you can buy instant relief in the form of a pill, potion or powder.

How did we get ourselves into this over-medicated mess? If you can back away from everyday actions and look at them with fresh eyes, some of the things we do don't make much sense— and in fact, have gotten us in big trouble. We got off track because no one taught us this formula:

$$RD + RE = SF$$
(Right Diet + Right Exercise = Senior Fitness)

Most people already recognize the need to consume a "proper diet" and get "some exercise." Many people think that they are doing just that by switching from eating red meat to chicken and fish, and getting out for a little walk once in a while. They then wonder why they still have high cholesterol, high blood pressure, aches and pains, diabetes, osteoporosis, and many of the other afflictions affecting people over fifty years old. At that point, they visit their doctor. The doctor listens to their complaints and their failed attempts at remedies, turns to the prescription pad (sometimes I think that MD stands for "more drugs"), and writes out a list of drugs for the patient to take. Both the patient and doctor are now on the same page—believing that drugs are necessary to treat these symptoms. Indeed, many of us don't feel we've got our money's worth from a doctor unless we walk out of the office with a prescription and a promise in hand. What is tragic is that these afflictions are almost always preventable and reversible.

THE RIGHT DIET AND RIGHT EXERCISE

You need to know up front one major premise of this book: what I consider the "right diet" is a whole-food vegan diet. A vegan diet is one that contains no meat, dairy, or eggs. You should also know that by "right exercise" I mean daily, vigorous, and sweaty exercise. Both of these ideas sound radical, I know. However, bear with me and I will show you in this book why it would be radical *not* to adopt this diet and exercise regimen.

Here's a snapshot of the problem: Of the top ten causes of death in this country, almost all, to one extent or another, are related to a meat-centered diet and a sedentary lifestyle. For those of you reading this who feel that veganism and vigorous exercise are too much, I have only one question about your current diet and exercise routine: "*How's it working for you?*" If your answer is that you've never felt better, that all your health indicators are fine, and that you're not on any medication and don't foresee any need to be on medication, then you can put this book down. If the answer is "Not very well," then read on.

GETTING OLDER DOESN'T NECESSARILY MEAN GETTING SICKER

You will frequently hear people complaining about their aches and pains and conclude that they are a necessary concomitant of aging. Even their physicians will sympathize and say, "What do you expect? You're getting older." Many of you have already heard "Well, let's face it, you're not a spring chicken anymore!" If you've been told that "It's just your age" or that "You'll just have to learn to live with it," here's an alternative thought. The most common diseases affecting older people are almost entirely related to lifestyle. In each of the following chapters, you will read how both diet and exercise can affect these most common (in this country, anyway) diseases or conditions.

If you eat the foods most Americans eat, you'll get the diseases most Americans get. Heart disease, cancer, strokes, diabetes, obesity, arthritis, osteoporosis, dementia, hypertension, and frailty are generally considered part and parcel of getting older. These conditions are highly prevalent only in Western societies and rare in non-industrialized societies. That should tell us *all* something, but somehow we're missing the message. Most of these chronic degenerative diseases are preventable and reversible by following the Senior Fitness equation described in this book.

UNNECESSARY DRUGS

We also need to remember that there is a considerable risk that the drugs themselves will cause a whole new set of problems, especially when you have multiple prescriptions. Drug interaction is a major killer in this country.[1] Even aspirin, which has generally been considered safe for many years, has according to a recent study been found to put you at an overwhelming eighty-six percent increased risk of pancreatic cancer, one of the worst types of cancer, when taken daily.[2] (If you have been prescribed aspirin, you should not stop taking it without the approval of your physician, because the benefits may outweigh the risks. In fact, do not make *any* changes in prescription drugs without the knowledge of your personal physician.)

What you may not know, however, because nobody can make money off it, is that, according to a Scottish study comparing vegetarians and nonvegetarians, if you eat lots of fruits and vegetables, the levels of salicylic acid (the active ingredient in aspirin) in your blood will go up and inflammation will decrease.[3] The foods with the highest salicylic acid content are broccoli, chili peppers, tomatoes, cucumbers, sweet potatoes, blackberries, cherries, cranberries, dates and plums. These foods won't eat up your stomach lining, either, the way aspirin does.

The average sixty-five-year-old with diabetes and hypertension takes *nine* different drugs,[4] putting him or her at risk for drug interactions that can be horrifying—and fatal. One example is the cholesterol-lowering drug Baycol. The side effects of Baycol have been devastating for many patients and their families. Charles Young of Pinole, California began taking the prescription drug Baycol in March 2000 to reduce his cholesterol. Soon he began suffering from leg pains, which rapidly worsened to the point that he could not walk. Young's physician did not recognize the cause of the leg pains and prescribed only pain medication. Young's condition continued to deteriorate, and soon he was admitted to the hospital. Within twenty-four hours of his admission, Young experienced complete kidney failure and was put on kidney dialysis. Subsequently, Young suffered a severe heart attack and died on May 24, 2000. The drug has since been withdrawn.[5] There are hundreds of thousands of deaths just as horrifying as this one that have been documented. More recently, the drug Vioxx was withdrawn from the market when it was discovered that it had caused 27,000 heart attacks,[6] and it was found that heartburn and ulcer medications such as Nexium, Prilosec, and Pepcid put people at almost double the risk of contracting pneumonia.[7] Again, a change in diet and an effective exercise program can reverse these conditions and eliminate the need for almost all of these drugs.

Painkillers, appetite suppressants, antacids, statins, antiinflammatories, antihistamines, laxatives, fiber supplements, antibiotics, antidepressants, hormones, sexual stimulants, and even alcoholic beverages: With the exception of antibiotics, most of these drugs treat the *symptoms* of a condition and do not do a thing to eliminate the cause, leaving the disease condition to progress because the cause has not been corrected. It's analogous to fighting fires by disabling the fire alarms. Indeed, in the case of antibiotics, if the immune system is functioning properly, there may be no need for them, either.

What most drugs do is merely *disable the body's "alarm" system*, the desperate calls for help that the body is sending out. Unfortunately, covering up the symptoms allows the disease condition to progress unabated. Then, as we have seen, these drugs have their own side effects, which are frequently covered up by yet another prescription drug.

In each of the disease conditions listed above, there are standard drug therapies administered by medical professionals. For example, for heart disease, patients may be given a statin, a cholesterol-lowering drug that they are told they will need to take for the rest of their life but which is not without serious side effects. For cancer, doctors usually prescribe chemotherapy and radiation, though there is little evidence that these procedures extend life. For diabetes (usually Type 2), patients are given insulin or, if it's not too late, glucose-lowering drugs. Patients are usually not told that a lifestyle change can reverse the diabetes. For arthritis, doctors offer anti-inflammatories or Cox II inhibitors (the latest drugs on the market), again, with possibly significant side effects. A change in diet may eliminate all joint pain. For osteoporosis, patients may be given Fosamax, a drug that stops the action of the osteoclasts (the bone cells that make way for new bone), and thereby gives the impression that bone is getting stronger. Such a regimen ignores the fact that the bone is getting more brittle and that the drug may be burning a hole in your esophagus. And they are often not told that exercise will strengthen bones.

For constipation, you may take Ex-Lax, Correctol and Metamucil, when simply adding fruits and vegetables to the diet will take care of the problem. For hemorrhoids, there is Preparation H, the need for which is also caused by lack of fruits and vegetables in the diet. For dementia, doctors may prescribe antidepressants that can make memory even worse. For hypertension, diuretics or "water pills" can lower blood pressure by causing increased urination; however, they also can cause an imbalance of electrolytes.

For menopause, women were for years prescribed powerful *horse* estrogens that led to so many heart attacks, strokes, blood clots, cancers of the breast and uterus, asthma, and hearing loss that automatic prescriptions were finally stopped for post-menopausal women.[8] Now doctors are prescribing Prozac. In addition, frailty might be treated with potent steroid hormones.

In each of these cases, patients are rarely told of an alternative: that a change to a vegan diet and an effective exercise program can help them avoid these drugs by eliminating the *cause* of the disease.

So, let's move on to an outline of the first component of my diet and exercise program: the diet.

CHAPTER 2

THE RIGHT DIET

O<small>PEN THE PANTRY</small> doors of most kitchens and you'll find lots of cans, jars, cardboard boxes, and plastic-wrapped packages of refined, processed foods. Open the refrigerator and freezer doors and you'll discover all kinds of dairy and animal products. (These animal products *must* be kept refrigerated to slow down the bacteria's rate of multiplying, which would spoil these products, leading to food poisoning and death.) Of the few plant foods in the typical kitchen, fruits and vegetables, you will find that they have been boiled, peeled, salted, sugared, chemicalized, sometimes radiated, and put into glitzy containers (for which you pay a pretty price). These foods often barely resemble their natural state.

Most foods in the typical American kitchen are animal foods, which are the true "weapons of mass destruction" because they kill more than 400,000 Americans every year.[1] This book will show you how these weapons work.

THE "BOOMERS" ARE COMING

Nature is kind to children in that they can get away with all kinds of dietary indiscretions and still survive to the age of reproduction. Once that age is passed, however, the debts must be paid. The process of heart disease, for example, starts in children as young as two years of age when fatty streaks start appearing in their arteries,[2] but they may not have a heart attack until they reach fifty years of age. There is an alarming epidemic of obesity in children[3] that will be progressively harder to reverse as they get older. Because of the "Baby Boom," there are millions of people turning fifty every year and, with that, entering the period of their lives that is most expensive in terms of medical intervention.

It doesn't have to be this way. If people would be willing to make some changes in their lifestyles, they could avoid almost *all* of these afflictions. Unfortunately, the problem is that they are not getting the medical advice they need to support their making the necessary changes. Another part of the problem is that most people view giving up their "favorite" foods and having to "(ugh!) exercise" as a tremendous sacrifice, and many think they'd rather give up some longevity in favor of what they view as "quality of life." Sadly, they don't know that the "quality" of their lives can improve way beyond their wildest dreams. The secret is: **You can learn to love what's good for you**. The purpose of this book is to show you how to do this.

The first thing we need to do regarding diet and the race for life is to understand how our bodies work in terms of the nutrients we put in them and how we move those nutrients around. I promise to do a lot of explaining so that you'll see for yourself how and why this program works. We're not going to wait decades while the researchers dig out and continue to debate these "truths," because it might be too late for you or someone you know. Besides, you risk nothing by starting this program now, and you have a lot to lose by waiting the ten years or so before this advice becomes "mainstream." (Even then, there'll probably be some doctors and diehards still waiting for confirmation. Look how long it took cigarette-smoking physicians to stop advertising cigarettes! I can remember the ads that quoted doctors claiming that smoking was soothing to the throat, the "T Zone." There were also doctors who claimed that smoking was good for pregnant women. The tobacco industry is still fighting those who claim that secondhand smoke is bad for you.) Know also that very little nutrition is taught in medical school, and most of what is taught is parenteral (or "outside the intestine") nutrition, which instructs doctors on how to keep a person alive through IV (intravenous) feedings. These feedings provide only salt and sugar, which is hardly what anyone would call good nutrition.

HOW TO SAVE YOUR LIFE

Let's talk about your body. Take a look at your hands. You're looking at just a few million of the 73 trillion[4] or so cells that make up "you"—and every single one of them depends on you. We're going to talk about the care you are giving those cells that make up that body of yours.

Our body is like an automobile, except that none of us has an O & M (operations and maintenance) manual to make sure we run the machine properly. Nobody is sure, for instance, about the correct octane fuel needed to maintain our bodily machine, beyond the initial fuel of our mother's breast milk. Maybe we are really diesel engines but we keep going to the same old service station and getting the same old gasoline in our tanks. When it comes to oil viscosity, maybe we should be using forty-weight but all that's available is five-weight. You look at your car's body, and you can't see that yucky sludge that's building up in the engine. You look at your hands, and you can't see that yucky sludge that's building up in your circulatory system and around your heart, either. Make no mistake—that sludge is there if you're eating the Standard American Diet (SAD).

You probably already know enough about anatomy and physiology to be aware that our body consists of a closed-circuit system with the heart as the pump (contracting an average of seventy-two times a minute), which pushes our blood to all parts of the body—to each of those 73 trillion cells. The arteries that lead directly out of the heart are very large and they keep branching off, getting smaller and smaller until, as capillaries, they are barely as wide as one blood cell. From there, they reverse direction and start joining up again, getting larger and larger as veins, and the blood cells make their way back up to the heart to start their journey all over again. Now, if you had a transparent body, you could see the heart beating and squirting blood out with each beat. Not surprisingly, given its function, it is absolutely *critical* that the heart is nourished, and this is what the coronary arteries do.

CHOLESTEROL

OK, so far, so good. Now, let's look at the fuel we're putting in our tank. The components of food consist of carbohydrates, protein, fat, vitamins, and minerals. If the food we eat is of plant origin, we are also getting phytonutrients ("phyto" means "plant") and fiber. If the food we eat is of animal origin, we are adding cholesterol but no phytonutrients and fiber. Cholesterol is not really a nutritional component because it can't be metabolized and has no calories. The worst part of cholesterol, however, is that our bodies have no efficient way to get rid of any excess.[5] If your diet is all whole plant foods, there will be no cholesterol in it. Furthermore, plant foods are usually low in fat and have no saturated fat. They will also contain lots of fiber. Mounting evidence suggests that this is perfect nutrition—everything we need with the exception of B-12 (which will be discussed later), and nothing we don't need. Simply put: Hearts thrive on plant foods, and clog up on animal foods.

Now, look at the animal products some of us use as food. While these may give us some of the nutrients we need for a healthy body, they don't provide them in the right proportions—and they give us a whole lot of what we don't need along with what we do. There is cholesterol in every single cell of every single animal, since it is a component of animal cell walls. The high-protein diet of the type that is very popular now (if that diet consists mainly of animal products) offers too much protein, very few carbohydrates, too much saturated fat (which increases the viscosity of the blood), too much iron, and no fiber at all. In fact, an essential difference between plants and animals is that a plant's cell walls are made of fiber and animals' cell membranes are made of cholesterol. That's why it is impossible to avoid eating cholesterol as long as you're eating any animal product. One way to remember this is: **Fiber is to plants as cholesterol is to animals**.

You may have heard that a high blood cholesterol level is not a good predictor of heart disease because (the reasoning goes) it appears that many people with "normal" cholesterol have heart attacks. The fallacy here is with the term "normal." "Normal" in this country is 210 mg/dl.[6] "Normal" levels in rural China and among the Tarahumara people of Mexico, however, are 120[7] and 125,[8] respectively. Heart attacks and coronary artery disease are virtually nonexistent among these populations, but are very common in this country with average cholesterol levels of 210 mg/dl. Now can you see why people in this country with so-called "normal" cholesterol are still having heart attacks? Can you see why drug companies are trying to get everybody on their cholesterol-lowering drugs? Even *they* recognize that our cholesterol levels are too high, and they see a potential bonanza.

What do people do about their diet when they are told their cholesterol levels are high? They do what I thought I had to do: switch from "red meat" to "chicken and fish." They discover, however, that their cholesterol stays the same. They and their doctors then conclude that they "tried the diet but it didn't work." The diet didn't work because there's just as much cholesterol in chicken and fish as there is in beef.[9] Although the cholesterol content in animal foods is not the only factor in blood cholesterol levels, and switching to chicken and fish will slightly lower the amount of saturated fat in your diet, you will not substantially reduce your risk of a heart attack. Here, half-truths and misinformation serve to disguise a viable method of reducing cholesterol levels without using drugs. In this scenario, only the patient loses.

This is why we need fiber, which we'll discuss in more detail later, but for now know that our bodies' intestinal systems need lots of fiber to maintain their operational efficiency. Our bodies don't need anyone else's cholesterol because our own livers produce all we need. In fact, any cholesterol that we eat from animals is automatically excessive, automatically *beyond* what our bodies need. The damage done by this cholesterol starts when it builds up inside our arteries. This process, we have noted, starts in children as young as two years of age when eating the SAD diet.

When the tiny arteries have even a thin layer of cholesterol and fat deposited in them and become inflamed, they have the potential to block off the flow of blood. This process occurs in many places throughout the body. If the blockage is in the coronary arteries, we have a heart attack, which can leave part or all of the heart muscle dead, and we may need coronary bypass surgery. If we do not change our diet, and continue eating animal products, the buildup of cholesterol and fat continues—except now, for reasons that doctors have yet to determine, at an accelerated rate. If the blockage is in the arteries leading to the brain, we have a stroke. Because we cannot yet perform brain bypass surgery, stroke damage can be devastating. If they are not killed, victims can be left paralyzed, with memory loss, impaired speech, and loss of other functions. If the blockage is to the kidneys, we have to go on dialysis for the rest of our days. If the blockage is to the big toe or lower leg, we get gangrene and have to have that part amputated.

THE NOT QUITE INVISIBLE PROCESS

Most of the damage that occurs to our arteries through poor diet and no exercise occurs invisibly, and we don't know what is happening until a crisis like one of the ones listed above occurs. There is, however, one graphic exception.

By the age of sixty, one man in four is impotent,[10] mainly because the identical process that goes on in the heart also goes on in every part of the body, including the penis. In my experience, people (especially men) have a hard time picturing their coronary arteries closing, but they sure can picture this! Because we haven't yet figured out a way to do genital bypass surgery, medical science has come up with a number of solutions to work around the problem of blood being blocked to the penis— Viagra, penile implants, injections, rings, and pumps. However, they all seem to leave a lot to be desired!

Unfortunately, that's not the end of the bad news. Some urologists claim that if a man lives long enough, he *will* get cancer of the prostate. Of men over the age of forty-five, one in five in this country already have cancer cells in their prostate gland.[11] The good news is that men living in countries who don't eat the way we do have a much lower risk of cancer of the prostate.[12]

TWO HOURS TO SAVE YOUR LIFE

My visit to Dr. John McDougall after I had been diagnosed with cancer changed my life. It took me *less than two hours* to learn most of the dietary information that's in this book. What I then found was overwhelming evidence in the implication of *all* animal foods—that just taking the skin off chicken or buying water-packed tuna wouldn't help, and that even skim milk wasn't good for you, either.[13] So I gave them up—just like that! It's so easy when you can *see* the cancer, or *see* the blocked arteries, or whatever body system is showing up damaged first. I say "first" because the damage is being done to all of our 73 or so trillion cells—it just takes a while for you to see it.

This is only an outline of the diet. (You can read more about diets in Chapter 5.) Throughout this book you will have a good idea of what I eat and where I get my energy. Now let's discuss the second component of my health regimen: the right exercise.

CHAPTER 3

THE RIGHT EXERCISE

ALONG WITH PUTTING the proper fuel in our bodies, the other half of the program for taking proper care of our bodies is exercise. This is the mechanism that acts as a booster for the heart—a secondary pump to increase the oxygen to those 73 trillion cells and expedite the removal of the waste products our body is constantly creating.

Here again, we have to look at motivation. How do we get motivated to exercise? I've talked to dozens of doctors who say they invariably tell their patients to get more exercise. Yet how many doctors exercise themselves? Some people complain about the *pain* of exercising. I can tell you this: *The pain of discipline is nothing compared to the pain of regret!*

As a former logistician in the field of acquisition logistics, designing and selecting components based on life cycle costs for the Air Force's F-16 aircraft, I used to say, "You can pay me now or you can pay me later." It's the same with our lives. You *will* give up eating animal products—the only question is *when*. Will you do it before more damage is done or will you wait for the wake-up call, which in the case of most heart attacks is too late?

"Pay me now or pay me later" also applies to exercise. The other day as I was finishing up my swim, I saw an older man dragging one leg and one arm—the characteristic walk of a stroke victim. He walked up to the chin-up bars, picked up his right hand with his left, laid it on the bar, wrapped the fingers around it, and did what he could in the way of little pull-ups. *What a sad example of "pay me later,"* I thought. You can do it now willingly or you can wait until a physical therapist prescribes it as rehabilitative therapy.

My secret is that if you make exercise fun, it's a whole lot easier to get it done. Now, you need to know that when I talk exercise, I'm pretty heavy duty. I have completed the Ironman Triathlon six times, have run sixty-seven marathons and over 100 smaller triathlons, and have won nearly a thousand first place trophies. While I agree that not everybody has to go out and do a triathlon or run a marathon to be healthy, I want to remind you that I believe *you could if you wanted to.* After all, at one point, I was your typical sedentary couch potato, eating animal products twenty-one times a week, with high cholesterol and blood pressure levels. I had arthritis—and that was *before* I got breast cancer. Once I understood what was happening, once I "saw" the process inside my body, it was easy—and I just want to show you how easy it can be, too.

Exercise is such powerful therapy that it can also be a cure for obesity. Americans are now the fattest, sickest people on earth, and I believe it's because we are putting the wrong fuel in our bodies and not putting fun in our exercise. Exercise is the closest thing you will find to the "Fountain of Youth." It even boosts the power of the immune system and is the most effective stress reliever I know of (I'll talk more about this later).

All of this is powerful medicine. In fact, I know a good many MDs—like John McDougall, Michael Klaper, William Harris, Neal Barnard, Robert Kradjian, Terry Shintani, Caldwell Esselstyn, and Michael Greger—whose patients get this prescription instead of therapy such as drugs, surgery, and radiation. If our health-care systems would implement this kind of medicine, we'd eliminate most cases of premature death, and save billions of dollars in needless health-care costs.

You will see and feel the difference in a very short time! Then maybe we could make the headlines: "No more heart disease, cancer, diabetes, arthritis, and obesity! New health program delivers more energy, better looks, deeper sleep, and lots, lots more!"

A SECOND CHANCE AT LIFE

Don't you sometimes wish you could start life all over again? Look at how much you've learned, how many mistakes you could now avoid, and what you could contribute to the world, if only you were given a chance!

Well, you are now being given the chance. What follows in this book is not difficult—although it may seem so at first. So many people see the light at the end of the tunnel and convince themselves that it's a train! I don't know how many times I've started a race—the starting line of the Ironman Triathlon, for example—thinking that this was going to be impossible for me to complete, that perhaps I hadn't trained enough, or that, at the very least, it was going to be very painful, if not agonizing, and certainly not fun. But in each of the thousand-plus races I've done, I've crossed the finish line, looked back and thought, *I can't believe it was that easy! Wow, am I glad I showed up for the race!* In fact, in more than 900 of those races, I've earned a gold medal. Taking home "hardware" makes exercise even more rewarding. I'll tell you another one of my secrets right now.

Lots of times I've collected a first place trophy because I was the only one in my age group. That's when I learned that eighty percent of winning is just showing up; eighty-five percent is showing up on time; ninety percent is showing up on time and being well trained; ninety-five percent is showing up on time, well trained, and having set the goal of completing the race; and 100 percent of winning is showing up on time, well trained, having winning as the goal, and just going out and doing it!

Although lots of people have certain handicaps or disabilities, I think anyone can benefit from this program. When you've seen paraplegics in wheelchairs alongside you in a race, you know you have no excuse for not showing up. When you develop that kind of commitment, you know you're doing it because the rewards are that great. I've heard people call this program "radical." There's very little that's "radical" about what I do; what *is* "radical" is what modern, industrialized life has done to us and our bodies. "Radical" is sawing open people's chests to reroute their heart's blood supply or putting them on dangerous drugs for the rest of their lives. It's time to regain control!

EXERCISE IS NOT ENOUGH!

At the time of my diagnosis, I had been a runner for fourteen years. I didn't know it then, but I was extremely fit but not healthy. This came about because, apart from my reading, one of my "obsessions" was my daily morning run. Way back in 1968, a medical doctor named Kenneth Cooper had written a book entitled *Aerobics*,[1] a word I'd never seen before, since Dr. Cooper had just coined it.

The word jumped out at me as I was walking past a bookshelf, and, being curious, I picked up the book and started thumbing through it. It seemed that every chapter addressed an ailment that plagued me: backaches, constipation, insomnia, fatigue—even flat feet! Anything that could cure all these problems promised a lot, so I bought the book, took it home and read it in one sitting. At almost two o'clock in the morning, I put it down, rolled over and fell asleep. When I awoke at the ungodly hour of five A.M., I felt strangely energized. I jumped out of bed, went to my closet, found an old pair of tennis shoes, put on a pair of cuffed Bermuda shorts (that was the closest I could come to running shorts back then) and a t-shirt, and went out the door for my first run.

I can remember how weird it felt. I hadn't done any running since I was a kid. My muscles were doing something they'd only have done if I were being chased by some sinister character. However, in another strange sense, it felt good to be so physical. I was breathing hard and having a little trouble getting my breath, so I slowed down. It never got uncomfortable enough for me to stop, though.

At the end of my street, about a half a mile, I turned around, determined to run all the way back. Besides, I was running out of time and had to get to work. When I got back to the house, I had this healthy, pink flush on my face, my muscles felt invigorated, and the sweat I had worked up was evidence that I'd really accomplished something.

The next morning I awoke at the same time and did it again. I was a little sore from the day before, but not enough to deter me. In fact, this time it was a little easier.

As I continued my daily morning runs, I could feel my strength increasing, my energy level going up. Best of all, however, I could eat more. In fact, I *had* to eat more to keep from losing too much weight. This had *never* happened to me before!

I started sleeping more soundly, dropping off to sleep as soon as my head hit the pillow and sleeping all the way through without awakening. When I'd wake up in the morning, I was pleasantly surprised to find that my bowels worked immediately. *That* had never happened before, either! I'd been constipated my whole life. Every morning from then on, just like clockwork, my bowels functioned. It was almost as if they knew they had to do their thing now, because later I'd be on the road!

The flab that was starting to appear on my thighs disappeared, and now there was muscle definition in both my upper and lower legs. The backaches that had plagued me, almost landed me in the hospital under a surgeon's knife—a myelogram (back x-ray) showed I had two "ruptured discs"—soon disappeared. Nobody had told me that most backaches have a dietary and exercise component and that back pain can have the same cause as chest pain—lack of oxygen. I also noticed that when I walked on a wet surface and looked back, the footprints that I left even had arches. The physical changes in my body were very obvious in a matter of weeks, and I loved every one of them—especially the one about the thighs, which Dr. Cooper hadn't even mentioned.

Then there was the matter of stress. At that point in my life, I had two adolescent kids (need I say more?) and a demanding job, and I was trying to finish up my doctoral degree. I was frequently "stressed out" and had no idea how to handle it. Those poor people around me, especially my kids, suffered the consequences. But with the morning runs, I found that it was a perfect time to process "mental data." I'd go over in my mind the things that would come up. I'd rehash conversations that had left me frustrated and annoyed and think of all the things I *should* have said. I'd visualize a different outcome and feel much better. The creative juices got cooking and I'd come up with a whole list of what I was going to accomplish that day.

By the time my run was finished, I could hardly wait to get started with my day. With the additional energy that running gave me, I was able to accomplish more, being far more efficient than I'd been before. So not only was I sleeping better at night, but my days got better, too.

I've been running ever since, and, as you will see later on in this book, it has enabled me to recover more quickly from some of the accidents I've had and some of the health setbacks I've experienced over the last two decades. What you need to know right now, however, is that you can do it—and later I'll show you how. Before that, however, let's examine what aging actually means.

CHAPTER 4

WHAT IS AGING?

D ID YOU KNOW that scientists really don't know what aging is? Gerontologists don't even know how many genes are involved in aging—with estimates ranging from very few to thousands. We do know that telomeres at the ends of chromosomes play some sort of a protective role, and that each cell type has its own built-in biological clock.[1] As research has progressed, however, researchers have discovered that symptoms previously thought to be due to "aging" have turned out to be due to either disease or disuse.

Look at the two most common causes of death in this country, heart disease and cancer. Because they are strongly correlated with age, they were at first thought to be part of the aging process. Back in the 1950s, however, it was noted that other countries had almost zero rates of heart disease. During the Korean War, when autopsies were performed on young soldiers killed in action, it was found that Korean soldiers had whistle-clean coronary arteries, whereas the arteries of young American soldiers were clogged with plaque.[2] Further research showed that eating high-fat, high-cholesterol foods caused the coronary artery blockage and that changing to a low-fat vegan diet reversed it. Dr. Dean Ornish proved this could be done, adding meditation to reduce stress, exercise, and group support to ensure success.[3] Dr. Caldwell Esselstyn, Jr. did it with diet supported with added statins.[4] Those findings definitively eliminated "aging" as a cause of heart disease, and to most people looking at the data the evidence pointed quite clearly to diet as the major factor in heart disease.

What about cancer? When epidemiologists started noting different rates of different cancers in different countries, they discovered, for example, that breast cancer was practically nonexistent in countries where no one could afford to eat meat. Moreover, in those countries where meat was so affordable it could be eaten three times a day, breast cancer rates were the highest.[5] The same was, and is, true of colon and prostate cancer.[6] These were examples of diseases previously thought to be caused by "aging," and although you can't conclusively prove a cause-and-effect relationship by epidemiological studies, I think the evidence clearly points to diet as the culprit. The saddest part is that as developing countries are able to afford more meat, their cancer rates are rising.

Our seniors are thought to lose bone mass and muscle inevitably as they age, simply in the natural process of getting older. You can read in many textbooks that the rate of bone loss is, on average, one percent per year, and that muscle loss is ten percent per decade of life but accelerates to fifteen percent after age fifty.[7] You will lose at least eight to ten ounces of muscle per year if you don't do something to counteract that. What we now know is that anyone of *any* age will lose bone *if* he or she doesn't put adequate stress or loading on the bone.[8] A good example of this is when you put someone on complete bed rest or when you launch very fit astronauts into outer space where they don't even have gravity pulling on their bones. In both cases, they soon become so weak that they cannot even stand or walk.

LONGEVITY UNDER IDEAL CONDITIONS

Patricia Blanchette, MD,[9] a gerontologist, jokes about her patient population that she sends them back to their pediatrician if they are younger than eighty; she wants to study the "really" old ones. She has stated that every sign or symptom of "aging" that she has looked at has turned out to be due to either *disease* or *disuse*. Cataracts, glaucoma, and macular degeneration, for example, are not due to aging but instead seem to be correlated with a low intake of leafy green vegetables. Ovarian and testicular cancers have been correlated with a high intake of dairy products. Bone and muscle loss is due primarily to disuse. Brain and memory loss is from both disease and disuse. Dr. Blanchette claims that if we could isolate the heart, lungs, liver, or kidneys, for example, and put them in ideal laboratory conditions, they would last for at least two hundred years. It's the abuse we subject them to that causes them to first falter and then quit functioning completely.

Picture, if you will, a hospital nursery full of newborns. They are as similar to each other as they will ever be, regardless of the different genetic permutations that each baby inherits. In fact, you could take nurseries from all over the world, and it would still be true: Regardless of race and ethnicity, babies are as similar to each other as they ever will be.

It's what happens to us from that time on, after we leave the nursery, that causes the individual divergence. Some babies get the tremendous advantage of breast feeding, while those who are fed formula don't get the immunities that their mothers have developed. (There are, of course, many more advantages to breast feeding that we won't go into here.) Then there is the wide range of diets and lifestyles that are available to the different cultures. Chinese children are fed very differently from American children. Many African kids run—not walk but run—six or eight miles to and from school every day, whereas American kids *may* ride a bike, if they are not driven by bus or car. These differences generally persist and even increase throughout our lives. At the end of our lives, we are as different as we have ever been—and it's all due to lifestyle.

As researchers tease out the information relating to causes of death and apply them to populations, they are predicting that life expectancy will increase. There are many demographers who suggest that within the next twenty-five years our life expectancy will increase by up to forty years. According to John Wilmoth, PhD, an associate professor of demography at the University of California, Berkeley, the human life span has been increasing more rapidly in recent decades.[10] As we learn to avoid "disease" and "disuse," we are then able to take better care of ourselves and go for the two hundred years theoretically allotted us.

What about all the other factors, however—those that are not related to disease and disuse? We know that smoking cigarettes and other tobacco products, the consumption of alcohol, and the use of illicit (and frequently "licit") drugs take a terrible toll on our lifespan.

A headline in the April 8, 2004 edition of *The Vancouver Sun* reads, "Booze is nearly as bad for us as tobacco: study findings expected to spark international debate about how to curb consumption." The journal *Nature* reported on the same day that, despite being a clear public health threat, alcohol has escaped the stark health warnings associated with tobacco. Because several studies showed that a drink a day reduced the risk of heart attacks in older men and women, alcohol was assumed to have some health benefits. However, the study's co-author, Jurgen Rehm, an addiction specialist at the University of Toronto, says alcohol abuse is a growing menace internationally. According to the study, "Even small amounts of alcohol increase the risk of injury and boost the chances of developing about sixty diseases, including several cancers, liver cirrhosis, and neuropsychological disorders." The other author of the study, Norman Giesbrecht, a senior scientist at the Centre for Addiction and Mental Health in Toronto, says the evidence that alcohol does almost as much harm as tobacco is "quite convincing." For the first time in twenty years, the World Health Organization plans for the next meeting of its annual World Health Assembly to have alcohol on the agenda, with a resolution calling for international action to reduce "alcohol-related harm." The article continues, "US, Canada, and Western Europe have six to eight percent of deaths linked to alcohol. On a global scale, public health experts have long worried about the millions of people drinking themselves to death."

I don't drink any alcohol, not even wine. This is not because I don't like to have fun and socialize (just ask my friends!), but because studies show and I know from my own life that alcohol is not optimal for long-term health. I had the opportunity to work for a short time at an Alcohol Rehabilitation Center and saw firsthand the damage that alcohol can do to the drinker, the family, society, and the health-care costs that affect us all.

A significant problem with having "just a little wine" is that you don't know until it is too late how much alcohol an individual can handle. Some studies, it is true, suggest that drinking a little wine is good for controlling heart disease, and I have no reason to dispute these findings. However, the diet and exercise program you are reading about in this book will control heart disease even better. I don't want you to read this book and think about all the things you can't do, because life is too short and there is too much fun to be had without feeling deprived. My plan is about living life to the fullest—feeling great, looking great, and living a long time. If you stop drinking and smoking and start exercising and eating healthfully, you will soon find that what you thought was too difficult, tiring, boring, or plain impossible not only makes you feel wonderful but is also fun.

THE ROLE OF STRESS IN AGING AND DISEASE

It has often been said that stress is at the bottom of most disease and the cause of most doctor's office visits—a factor in eighty percent of the visits, according to one study.[11] In fact, when a physician is at a loss to explain why you're sick, he or she is most likely to blame stress—a case of "when in doubt, blame the patient"! It used to be thought that stress caused heart attacks until the famous Framingham Study—a decades-long epidemiological study of citizens of Framingham, Massachusetts—showed that heart attacks were correlated with high cholesterol and diet. Stress used to be blamed for stomach ulcers, but now we know it is most often an infection caused by *H. pylori* bacteria. While stress does play a major role in health, it is not always bad.

It is stress that motivates us to do better—whether it's to learn a new skill, avoid difficult people, or seek relief from a symptom of an illness. It can be as basic as getting us to break into a run as we see a truck bearing down on us, or as common as our reaction when things don't go a certain way—usually "our" way. Our response to stress is to fight or to run, and that response is hard-wired into our brains. Such a response served us well in prehistoric times, but in today's society, such highly charged responses can cause damage to our internal organs.

The physiological effect of stress is to release a flood of hormones that cause our hearts to beat faster, our breathing to quicken, our pupils to dilate, and our muscles to tense—all getting us ready to fight or flee. When the cause of our stress is our boss or a spouse, for example, neither of these reactions will work effectively. That's when we get motivated to learn a new skill, or, frequently, how to negotiate. We also know that exercise is an excellent stress releaser, as it helps to dissipate the stress hormones and relax us. It is also during exercise that our brains go into a creative problem-solving mode, and that frequently provides the solution to our stressor. And, where do you find stress? Always between your ears! This implies that you can control your response to it and use it to your advantage, as a motivation to do better.

CULTURAL ASPECTS OF AGING— DO WE RESPECT OUR ELDERS?

One of the major problems relating to our elders is that we tend to "warehouse" them when they get difficult to handle. When problems such as frailty or a hip fracture due to osteoporosis occur, we tend to chalk it up to old age, write off the old folks and put them in a nursing home, where many of them are forgotten. It doesn't have to be this way. Maria Fiatarone has studied the effects of exercise on aging.[12] She went to a nursing home where the residents ranged in age from eighty-seven to ninety-five, wheeled in a variety of exercise equipment, ensured that the residents followed the protocol she developed, and found that at the end of six months the average increase in muscular strength was 175 percent. The residents gave up their crutches and walkers, could manage stairs, and had obviously increased their fitness levels to a great degree. That was the good news. The bad news was that at the end of the experiment, the equipment was wheeled out and the subjects lost their newly regained fitness. The lesson? Exercise has to be for life.

BOTTOM LINE—WHAT WE KNOW FOR SURE

Aging, if defined as the passage of time and an increase in our calendar years, *cannot* be stopped. Aging, if defined as the loss of strength, vitality, and the onset of chronic degenerative disease, *can* be stopped, or at least drastically slowed—and in many cases even reversed—by a low-fat, whole-food vegan diet and daily, vigorous exercise. It is up to you to choose which it's going to be.

CHAPTER 5

Why Diet Matters

THERE IS MORE confusion about diets than almost any other subject. Look at the number of "diet" books on any bestseller list and you will see what concerns people the most. Weight-loss books touting the "latest" diet sell millions of copies but have little more than disappointment to offer readers, who turn in desperation to the next promising weight-loss diet.

Part of the confusion comes from the fact that we read one day that certain foods are OK and other foods are not, while the next press release that comes out says just the opposite—that the food you thought was not OK is now not only not bad for you, but may even be good for you. How is anybody supposed to know, and who are we to believe? It's hardly surprising that some people just throw up their hands and say, "I'm going to eat what I want. Everybody's going to die someday, so I might as well just enjoy myself." Then, upon finding that their cholesterol, blood pressure, and weight have all risen even higher, they resolve to try another "diet."

The importance of one's dietary choices cannot be understated because of diet's role in virtually every disease known to humans (and even, believe it or not, the animals who live with them). On July 17, 2004, the US government declared obesity to be a "disease," just as cancer is considered a disease. This means that obesity will be covered by medical plans and more insurance and more drug money can be spent on obesity treatments and bariatric surgery. If obese people only had some basic nutrition information, it wouldn't be at all confusing. This is what we will try to do in this chapter—that is, provide enough basic nutritional information to allow anyone to make the right decisions about what to eat to stay healthy for a long life.

THE WHOLE STORY ABOUT "WHOLE" FOOD

If you were to look at any standard nutrition textbook, you'd see food broken down into several different categories. Macronutrients, for example, are the carbohydrates, protein, and fats. The micronutrients are the vitamins, minerals, phytochemicals, and antioxidants. Fiber is in a separate category because the body does not absorb it, and therefore it provides no nutrition. However, fiber plays a critical role in a healthy body. In fact, you can't be healthy without it.

Most people are well aware of the fact that carbohydrates, protein, and fat contain calories, but they are not sure of the roles these nutrients play in providing energy to our bodies, especially when they hear that "carbs make you fat." Carbohydrates and protein each have four calories per gram, while fat comes in at nine, more than double that amount. The average adult burns around 2,000–2,800 calories per day, but the range is wide because of the great variance between people in size and activity levels. If you were to do nothing but lie in bed every day, you might burn about 1,200 calories per day. Add to this the activities of daily living and you might burn 800 more calories. Strenuous exercise naturally burns even more.

Calories are a measure of heat and are subject to very rigid laws of physics. There is no getting around the fact that we need food to provide calories, and we need calories to survive and to exercise. We must balance the calories we consume in the form of food with the calories we expend throughout the day and night, or we will either gain or lose weight. This law of thermodynamics appears to be lost on some promoters of fad diets and the people who follow them. For example, those who lose weight on high-protein diets such as the Atkins diet generally do so because they take in fewer total calories, not because of any special characteristics of a high-protein diet.

CARBOHYDRATE MYTHS: "GOOD CARBS" AND "BAD CARBS"

There's been a surge in the promotion of high-protein, low-carb diets off and on for the past thirty years, although the first known example of such a diet was one created in 1863 by William Banting,[1] a British undertaker! Carbohydrates have been featured in these diets as the "bad guys" of nutrition for a number of reasons. Meanwhile, protein, while essential, has been overly promoted as the "good guy" in building muscle, losing fat, and, in general, promising near-miracles in the body. Carbs have also been implicated as a cause of diabetes since sucrose, or table sugar, is a carbohydrate, although a "simple" carbohydrate. There are different forms of sugar, and they are the building blocks of carbohydrates the way amino acids are the building blocks of proteins.

The variations in how carbohydrates enter the bloodstream have become measurable through the "glycemic index" (GI).[2] High-GI foods are supposed to be bad for you because they raise the blood sugar level quickly and therefore elevate insulin levels. Carrots, for example, have a high GI—although it's hard to conceive of how a carrot is "bad" for you simply because it gets into your bloodstream quickly. If you're running a marathon, for instance, you want that energy getting into your bloodstream as quickly as possible.

Promoters of low-carb, high-protein diets and/or diet pills have used the glycemic index to suggest that keeping carbohydrates out of the bloodstream is essential, but as you will see later when we discuss diabetes, carbohydrates are not the cause of high insulin levels. Of course, if you're not running marathons or indeed getting any exercise at all, carbs will be stacking up in the bloodstream, and that *is* bad! But even this formula is not as simple as it sounds. Meals are generally made up of several different foods, and proteins, fats, and fiber tend to slow down the absorption of one or two high-GI foods into the bloodstream, thus alleviating the build-up of insulin levels.

Carrots aside, foods that measure high on the glycemic index tend to be the processed, refined foods with lots of white sugar and white flour that nearly all nutritionists agree are "bad carbs"—the kind found in all "junk foods" and most fast foods. What is often overlooked in the flight from carbohydrates is that blood sugar, or glucose, is the fuel that the body runs on. In fact, it is the *preferred* fuel for the brain. While under extreme circumstances the body *can* use limited amounts of protein and fat for proper functioning, the *preferred* fuel for our bodies is, as any athlete will tell you, most definitely carbs. That's why "carboloading" parties are so popular before big races such as marathons and triathlons.

What most people don't know is that, just as there are "bad" carbs, there are also "good" carbs. Good carbs are those in their unrefined state—i.e., whole plant foods. (Apart from dairy products, there are essentially no carbohydrates in animal foods.) Good carbs include vegetables, fruit, whole grains, and beans.

Sometimes a food can be both a "good" carb and a "bad" carb. Take the potato, for instance. One hundred grams of plain, raw potato is seventy-six calories. When you boil the potato, it still contains seventy-six calories. Since baking a potato dehydrates it slightly, the calorie concentration goes up to ninety-three per hundred grams. However, if you cut the potato up into little "sticks" and deep-fat fry it, you have French fries, and the calorie count jumps to 274 per hundred grams. Eat a hundred grams of very thin, fried potato slices—that is, potato chips—and you're up to an amazing 568 calories. These are "bad carbs"! Most white flour products, pastas, and pastries fall into the category of "bad" carbs.

Another class of carbs—polysaccharides, such as cellulose—makes up the structural elements of cell membranes in plants and bacteria. Cellulose is fiber and has no calories for the human body. Glycogen, a chain of glucose molecules, is stored in the muscles of all animals (including us, of course) and is metabolized when we exercise. Insulin is the hormone secreted by the pancreas that keeps blood sugar levels steady and ushers carbs into the liver and muscles. When the liver and muscles can't hold any more, the carbs are turned into triglycerides or blood fats. When we consume too many calories, the excess is stored in the fat cells. Fat can be used as an energy source but it is more difficult to access than carbohydrate, as is protein. There will be more on this later in another chapter on exercise.

WHAT ABOUT PROTEIN?

Protein has long been praised as the "good guy" in the nutrition equation. Ever since early nutrition researchers discovered protein, it has been thought that since it was essential to life, one needed to consume a lot of it. In fact, it was generally assumed that the more protein one ate, the better. What is not as well known is that excess protein robs calcium from the bones, which can lead to osteoporosis and can also cause kidney stones.

One of the most frequent questions asked about vegan (strict vegetarian) or vegetarian diets, is "Where do you get your protein?" The simple answer is that there is more than enough protein in plant foods. Indeed, if you ate nothing but broccoli—say two thousand calories in a day—you would exceed each of the required essential amino acids by a substantial margin. Two thousand calories of broccoli would provide you with 3,043 mg of the essential amino acid methionine, for example, whose recommended daily allowance (RDA) is 425.[3] All the other essential amino acids exceed the minimums by even greater margins. This little dietary exercise holds true for every other vegetable. So, obviously, if you mix and match veggies according to your taste, you can't fail to get enough protein—as long as you get enough calories!

"GOOD" FATS, "BAD" FATS, AND "WORST" (TRANS) FATS?

You've probably heard that we need fat in our diet, but it's important to be aware of what kind of fat we're eating. The typical American diet consists largely of foods of animal origin, which are high in saturated fat. Saturated fats raise total cholesterol and low-density lipoproteins (LDLs) that clog arteries. Monounsaturated fats (found in olive oil and canola oil) in general lower LDLs without affecting the high-density lipoproteins (HDLs), the so-called "good cholesterol." Polyunsaturated fats are found in flaxseed and fish oil. Of the polyunsaturated fats, the best known are the "good" omega 6s (linoleic acid), which we usually get plenty of, and the other "good" fat, the omega 3s (linolenic acid), which we usually don't get enough of.[4,5] Not balancing omega 3s and omega 6s is very unhealthy for our brains and nervous system, because the myelin sheath, which insulates the brain and nervous system, is made of these good fats.

The imbalance between omega 3s and 6s can be taken care of

by avoiding refined, processed foods and adding a tablespoon of freshly ground flax seeds or a handful of walnuts daily to your diet. While fish oil is indeed a good source of omega 3 fatty acids, fish oil can be contaminated with pesticides, PCBs, mercury, and ciguatera toxin. Furthermore, fish don't create omega 3s themselves; they get them from eating chloroplasts in sea plants and algae. It should also be noted that, ounce per ounce, walnuts have more omega 3s than salmon.

Some medical authorities have counseled that flax seeds and flaxseed oil, while an important source of omega 3 fatty acids, are not as good a source of good fats as fish oil because the latter has eicosopentanoic acid (EPA) and docosahexaenoic acid (DHA), two fatty acids that our bodies can make given the essential omega 3 fatty acids. Others maintain that flax is sufficient because it provides adequate omega 3s. As I'm sure you're aware, however, studies are being produced all the time, and some of these contradict each other. What is essential is that you consume enough fat for your body to function properly. You should feel alive, full of energy, and, while your flesh should not be flabby (beyond the natural aging process), you should not be overly skinny. Again, monitor your body.

The "worst" fats are the trans fats that are found mostly in commercially prepared foods in the typical American diet. Trans fats, technically known as trans fatty acids (TFAs), are artificially made solid by heating oils under pressure in the presence of hydrogen and nickel, which makes the oil thicker by removing some of its chemical double bonds. This is usually done to extend the shelf life of foods. Trans fats are deadly because they elevate the levels of cholesterol in your blood even more than saturated fats, contributing more to your risk of heart disease. There is also evidence that trans fats interfere with the normal metabolism of essential fatty acids, leading to the disruption of the production of various hormones and blood clotting factors. As if that weren't bad enough, it is also suspected that trans fats trigger insulin resistance and increase your risk of developing Type 2 diabetes. They are very unnatural fats and can lodge long term (possibly forever) in the cell walls of your body.[6]

At least 30,000 premature heart disease deaths are caused each year by trans fatty acids. That's one death every fifteen minutes. On top of that, TFAs cause a far greater number of non-fatal but terrifying and damaging heart attacks. This information comes from one of the world's top authorities on nutrition, Dr. Walter Willett, Chairman of the Department of Nutrition at the Harvard School of Public Health and Professor of Medicine at the Harvard Medical School. Writing in the Harvard School of Public Health Report and *Eat, Drink and Be Healthy: The Harvard Medical School Guide to Healthy Eating*, Dr. Willett called trans fats "the biggest food-processing disaster in US history." Dr. Willett went on to say, "In Europe (food companies) hired chemists and took trans fats out. . . . In the US, they hired lawyers and public relations people. No one doubted trans fats have adverse effects on health, and still companies were not taking it out."

The US government has indicated that by the year 2006, food companies will have to tell us how many trans fats are in the food we're eating. In the meantime, you can estimate whether a product has trans fatty acids in it by looking for any ingredient called "hydrogenated" or "partially hydrogenated oil." This labeling, however, will not apply to restaurants. Toronto's *Globe & Mail* and CTV (Canadian Television) conducted a study and, without naming foods or restaurants, found that 100 percent of *all* the foods sampled had some amount of trans fatty acids in them. The National Academy of Sciences says the only safe intake of trans fats is zero.[7]

If you're eating a diet based on fruits and vegetables with lots of leafy greens, you'll get the right balance between the omega 3s (the "good" fats), very little of the "bad" fats, and no trans fats. For those who want to boost their levels of omega 3s, add a tablespoon of freshly ground flax seeds or walnuts, as mentioned above.

SO WHERE DO YOU GET YOUR CALCIUM?

The second most common question asked of vegans after "Where do you get your protein?" is "Where do you get your calcium if you don't consume dairy products or calcium pills?" As we did with protein, let's turn to broccoli. If you were to eat your 2,000 calories just in broccoli, you would consume more than 6,400 mg of calcium. Since the recommended daily amount is 1,200 mg, you can see that you would get more than enough calcium.[8] The same holds true of the other green vegetables. As long as you're consuming lots of greens, you generally won't need any calcium supplements, either.

THE DIFFERENCE BETWEEN PLANT FOODS AND ANIMAL FOODS

If you ever get confused as to whether a food is good or bad for you, there is a simple way to tell. Determine whether or not it is of plant origin. If it is, it's probably good for you. If it has a face, it's not good for you. This is because if your food had a face it probably also had a liver, and one of the basic differences between plant and animal foods is the presence of cholesterol in *all* animal products—including, of course, fish. We have already seen how cholesterol maintains the cell wall in animals and fiber maintains the cells of plants. We don't need to ingest cholesterol, because our own livers produce all the cholesterol we need for our own cell walls and to produce our hormones.

So what should be the ideal amount of cholesterol in our body—given that we know that high levels of cholesterol in the blood are a risk factor for heart disease, and that we decide not to add any extra cholesterol through eating animal products? Evidence from the Framingham Study suggests that we strive for a total serum cholesterol level of below 150 mg/dl, which renders us virtually immune to heart attacks, irrespective of HDL or LDL levels. HDL measurements are only important when you are at risk with a cholesterol reading higher than 150,[9] although there is an increasing tendency to target the LDL (the so-called "bad" cholesterol) at 100 mg/dl or below. While the Framingham Study showed that people with total cholesterol readings of 150 or below were virtually immune to heart disease, LDL readings get so much attention now because people eating the SAD diet are considerably above 150.

WHAT'S WRONG WITH DAIRY AND FISH?

I do not eat any animal by-products—eggs, butter, milk, yogurt, and even skim milk and powdered milk solids. My reason is that there are hormones, pesticides, and antibiotics—as well as cholesterol, of course—in all of these foods and absolutely no fiber. In addition, all these foods contain saturated fat, the so-called "bad fat."

Some people call themselves vegetarians when they still eat fish, as though the flesh of fish is different from, say, red meat. However, both are muscle, and all muscle contains fat and cholesterol. In fact, under a microscope one cannot tell the difference between muscle tissue samples from a cow, a fish, a pig, and a chicken[10]—and, because cholesterol is within the cell walls of all creatures that have a liver, beef and fish actually contain equal amounts of cholesterol. Studies differ on the fat content of different fish, and there are some "good" fats in fish. However, given the health consequences of the high concentrations of toxins in fish, and the fact that overfishing has left fish stocks decimated and caused the collapse of marine food chains throughout the world's oceans, you are far better off getting these fats in plant foods *without* the cholesterol and *with* the fiber.

WHY FIBER IS SO IMPORTANT

Fiber has no calories and is not absorbed in the intestinal tract, but it is an extremely important constituent in our diet.[11] We need fiber, or what used to be called roughage, to enable our intestines to move—a process technically called *peristalsis*. People who eat a low-fiber diet are frequently constipated and need to add fiber in the form of supplements. They may also need laxatives, suppositories or enemas, and are prone to hemorrhoids, appendicitis, and diverticula, which are outpouchings in the intestines that can get infected and cause diverticulitis. Diverticulitis can be serious enough to require surgery, yet it is easy to prevent simply by eating more plant foods. Fiber is also important in that it prevents the re-absorption into the intestines of cholesterol, fat, carcinogens, and hormones such as estrogen. It has been noted that heart disease and colon, breast and prostate cancers are much more common in people eating a low-fiber diet—in other words, a diet that does not contain many plant foods.[12]

WHAT CHOLESTEROL AND SATURATED FAT DO IN OUR BODIES

I have already examined the difference between so-called "good" cholesterol—high-density lipoprotein (HDL)—and "bad" cholesterol, low-density lipoprotein (LDL). I have suggested that if you do not consume cholesterol, your cholesterol levels should be normal, because your liver produces all the cholesterol your body needs. If your total serum cholesterol is below 150, your risk of the kinds of debilitating illness listed throughout this book is low. Your HDL as well as your LDL will also be low, because when you don't consume animal products you don't need a lot of HDL to carry away the "bad" cholesterol, since it's already at a healthy level.[13]

In this section, I will examine in more detail why excess cholesterol and saturated fats are bad for our bodies. High levels of cholesterol tend to clog arteries, causing inflammation and layers of plaque. This increases the risk of heart attacks, strokes, organ failure, and clots in the lower legs, which may even lead to amputation. Studies have shown that saturated and trans fats increase cholesterol levels even more than eating cholesterol directly. Both cholesterol and saturated fats are found in animal products and in processed, refined foods. Eating animal foods, with their saturated fat, also causes the red blood cells to get "sticky" and clump together, producing blood clots. Clots can be fatal when they travel through the body and get to the heart, brain, and lungs.[14]

There are three other factors that affect our risk of heart disease. Homocysteine is a by-product of protein metabolism and causes inflammation of the lining of the arteries. Homocysteine levels tend to be high when folic acid and B-12 levels are low. (Folic acid is found in leafy greens; B-12 we will get to shortly.)[15] The other factors that are tested for risk of heart disease and strokes are high levels of C-reactive protein, a measure of inflammation in the body,[16] and lipoprotein (a). These levels should all be low and can be monitored in blood tests. We'll talk more about this in the chapter on heart disease and strokes.

HOW TO LOWER CHOLESTEROL AS EFFECTIVELY AS STATINS

In the July 23, 2003 issue of the *Journal of American Medicine*, a study reported that the right diet would lower cholesterol as effectively as statins. Cyril Kendall, PhD, of the University of Toronto studied the evolution of our diets over the last ten to fifteen million years and concluded that we have always been primarily vegetarian.[17] He looked at present-day apes and found that the simian diet is still primarily vegetarian. The study took three groups of people and put them on controlled diets. The first group was put on a diet low in saturated fat. The second group ate a diet low in saturated fat plus a statin, and the third was given a diet with specific cholesterol-lowering foods. In just two weeks, all groups had lower cholesterol levels. However, the third group had a twenty-nine percent drop in cholesterol *without* drugs, compared to thirty-one percent with drugs.

The foods consumed in the third group consisted primarily of those foods that are most effective in lowering cholesterol, such as almonds, oat bran, legumes, and soy products. This group also had a lowering of the C-reactive protein levels, which, as mentioned, is a measure of the inflammatory process going on in the arteries. It was also noted that this third group found the diet enjoyable enough that they continued the diet even after the experiment ended. The results of this study demonstrate that cholesterol can be lowered as effectively with diet as with statins, so the drugs' side effects, such as constipation, gas, nausea, muscles aches and pains, fatigue, tendency to bleeding, and liver damage, can also be avoided. Statins are also very expensive and would need to be taken for life if people continued to eat foods with cholesterol.

THE RANGE OF DIFFERENT DIETS AND THE REASONS FOR THEM

You've probably heard of all kinds of diets that range from completely unrestricted to extremely restricted. The omnivore, for example, eats everything with no restrictions—except for the cultural taboos that all societies have. The omnivorous diet is the main diet of Westernized countries. Then there are several categories of vegetarian or plant-based diets. "Lacto-ovo vegetarians" do not eat meat but eat dairy and eggs. Some people who are vegetarian for ethical reasons find this diet acceptable because they believe that these foods do not cause the death of the animal (at least not immediately). Others may be lacto-ovo vegetarians because they believe that humans need the protein and/or calcium provided by the dairy and eggs.

The vegan eats only plant foods and frequently refrains from using any animal products such as leather, fur, and honey—depending on whether they are vegans for ethical or health reasons. I consider myself a vegan, not only because I truly believe that the diet has helped me keep healthy for all these years and has the power to create optimal health in everyone, but because I hate cruelty toward animals and people in all its forms. I have seen and read about what happens to many animals in intensive farming—commonly known as "factory farms"—and I do not want to be part of it. The best way I know not to consent to the routine cruelty and violence of modern-day farming practices is not to eat the animals treated in this way. This is one of the reasons, along with my concern for the environment and for maintaining optimum health, why I've chosen a vegan diet. Now, you certainly don't *need* to care about animal rights or the environment to eat healthfully. But it seems to me to be an added bonus for anyone seeking everyday fitness that you not only eat wonderfully vibrant and delicious food that keeps you healthy and strong, but you do not have to have an animal killed or degrade the environment to do so.

More and more people are becoming concerned about animal welfare and the horrible conditions that exist in factory farms. Many believe that slaughtering animals is inherently wrong—let alone cramming sentient creatures into filthy, feces-ridden cages, whether calves for veal or hens for eggs. While this book is about your health, and while I became a vegan because my life, literally, depended on it, I have read and seen enough over the years to know that I do not want to be part of an animal's death. Many great thinkers over the years, such as Socrates, Leonardo da Vinci, Mahatma Gandhi, and Albert Einstein have stated that killing and eating animals is morally wrong, and I have no problem being in that company! Indeed, it now seems strange to me when someone isn't disturbed by the wholesale killing of nine billion land animals each year in the United States. That's a lot of animals to kill to make us so sick.

Meat is not only bad for us on its own, but the mistreatment of animals has a direct bearing on the stress hormones in the meat. Growth and sex hormones are also added to the animal's food, or injected to get faster growth, while the rampant use of antibiotics is leading to the development of "superbugs" for which no antibiotic is effective. Food poisoning, which may masquerade as "stomach flu," is a growing threat to us all, but especially to children and older people whose immune systems may be compromised. Factory farms also create huge manure lakes that contaminate the aquifers, a major source of our drinking water. The grazing of cattle leads to the desertification of our lands. These are real problems that concern many scientists, medical professionals, and lay people.[18]

Another diet that is gaining in popularity is the raw food diet. This diet includes only uncooked vegetables and fruit, and excludes other categories of plant foods such as grains and legumes, either because they cannot be eaten raw or because they are not considered as nutrient-rich as fruits and vegetables, especially the leafy greens. Raw nuts and seeds may also be included in this category. I have been "raw" for four years now. In other words, my diet consists of eating mainly raw fruits and vegetables. Some doctors have suggested that a diet whereby whole grains and beans are not eaten daily will deprive the body of essential nutrients. Other doctors have suggested that a raw food diet is perfectly adequate. My advice, always, is to listen to your body and to seek the advice of as wide a range of nutritional experts as you feel comfortable with.

WHAT ARE PHYTONUTRIENTS?

A whole new exciting area of research is focused on phytonutrients ("phyto-" meaning "plant"). These are health-promoting, disease-preventing compounds that are found only in plant foods, and every plant has them. There are said to be hundreds, if not thousands, of them, and more are being discovered every day. Some of the most thoroughly researched phytonutrients are listed below.

Lycopene is a pigment that gives tomatoes, guavas, and watermelons their red color. A number of studies have linked it to lower risks of prostate cancer and heart disease.[19]

Lutein and zeaxanthin are classed as carotenoids and seem to protect against age-related changes occurring in the eyes—namely, cataracts and macular degeneration. The best sources of these phytonutrients are leafy greens and broccoli.

Anthocyanin is a cancer-fighting substance found in blueberries and blackberries.

Saponin appears to have a number of very positive roles in the body. It helps stimulate the immune system, slows growth of cancer cells, and blocks the absorption of cholesterol. It is found in legumes such as garbanzos and soybeans.

Tannins help reduce the risk of heart disease and are found in cranberries and green tea.

Lignans are very important in protecting against colon and breast cancer. They help lower estrogen levels by blocking reabsorption through the GI tract. Lignans are found primarily in flax seeds and whole grains.

Resveratrol is found in grapes and wine and is thought to be the substance in wine that lowers the risk of heart attacks. It's better to get your resveratrol from the grapes directly. Better yet, lower your risk of heart disease by changing your diet to avoid all animal products.

The best-known *isoflavones* are daidzien and genistein, which are beneficial primarily as estrogen analogues, since they are thought to block estrogen receptor sites. This in turn leads to a lowering in the risk of breast cancer and postmenopausal symptoms such as hot flashes. They are found in soy products such as tofu and miso.

Polyphenols are said to be helpful in preventing or reversing skin wrinkles. They also have a number of other healthful benefits. They are found in green tea.

Glyconutrients are immunity-boosting compounds that researchers have found to increase the ability of immune cells to fight infections. Some studies suggest that they can shorten the duration of an infection from a cold or flu. They are found in shiitake mushrooms.

Procyanidin is a compound that protects the heart by preventing blood platelets from forming clots. It's found in cocoa and chocolate (dark chocolate contains more cocoa than milk chocolate).[20]

There are many more phytochemicals that could be added to this list, and scientists are still discovering the benefits from the thousands of nutrients in fruits and vegetables. But we are still a long way from knowing all the benefits of these phytonutrients.

HOW TO HANDLE FOOD CRAVINGS

All of us get food cravings from time to time and, depending on what it is you're craving, it may be okay to give in to them. Our bodies may be signaling that we need a specific nutrient—or, as some, namely Neal Barnard, MD, have proposed, we may simply be addicted to the opioids found in some foods. It's hard to tell the difference sometimes. You can be sure, however, that if the craving is for chocolate or cheese, it's the opioids talking to you. If your craving is for watermelon, a nice, red, juicy apple, or a crunchy cucumber, indulge yourself; if, however, you crave chocolate or cheese, go for a healthy substitute such a carob treat or soy cheese. Don't do as I used to do—get rid of temptation by giving in to it. Get a healthy substitute, instead!

EATING WHAT OTHERS THROW AWAY

It will come as no surprise to you that we are a throwaway culture. However, it may be a surprise to some of you that along with the garbage and waste, we also unthinkingly throw some excellent food sources.

For example, watermelon seeds are very good sources of zinc and other minerals and fiber, but you have to be sure to chew them or else they go right through you. The same is true of flax seeds, but since they are so small, most people grind them. I hate to see seedless watermelons for a number of reasons (not the least of which is an objection to the trend toward genetically modified food, because I believe we are tinkering with the unknown), and missing the good taste of watermelon seeds is one of them. Grape seeds are getting harder to find as seeded grapes are increasingly replaced by insipid "seedless grapes"—while at the same time people pay good money to buy grapeseed extract in health food stores! Pumpkin seeds, citrus seeds and pith (the white part of the peel from oranges, lemons, grapefruit, tangerines, etc), tomato, cucumber, and bell pepper seeds are other examples of foods I like to eat.

Celery leaves are also thrown out as if they were inedible. As far as I'm concerned, the leaves are the best part and contribute to my intake of leafy greens. I have also shocked a number of people when they see me eat a whole hairy-skinned kiwi or mango complete with peel (make sure you are not allergic to mango peel before you try this). There are, of course, exceptions to eating seeds and peels, such as with papaya and cantaloupe. But, when you are preparing your fruits and veggies, watch for the best parts that sometimes get thrown away.

FOOD COMBINING AND YOUR IDEAL WEIGHT

Every decade, it seems, somebody decides that you should not eat protein with carbohydrates, or carbohydrates with fat, etc., because of the digestive enzymes in the stomach. I've never experienced any difficulty in mixing fruits and vegetables and, when you look at the logic of it, all foods as prepared by Nature come already combined with carbohydrates, protein and fat.

If you wonder what your ideal body weight is, you need to ask another question: How much body fat are you carrying? The standard measure of weight—the Body Mass Index (BMI)—is only a rough guide and does not tell you how much fat you are carrying. (This will be covered in more detail in the chapter on obesity.)

It used to be difficult to test for body fat percentage, but body fat testing scales are now readily available and fairly accurate. A male's body fat percentage should range from five to twenty percent and a female's from twelve to thirty percent. If you check some of the tables that come with body-fat testing equipment, you may find that the allowable body fat percentage increases with age. However, I believe that ideally you should not be gaining fat as you age. I'm old enough to remember that in the 1950s the rule for blood pressure used to be 100 plus your age. We now know that these numbers were too high, so the rule has been changed. The same situation occurred with cholesterol, when a measurement of 200 plus your age was once considered appropriate. It was noted that such high levels were conducive to heart attacks, and now we find a similar situation with body fat percentage. Aging should *not* increase blood pressure, cholesterol and body fat.

You want as much lean body mass—that is, muscle and bone—as possible. The best way to increase muscle and bone is exercise, which will be covered in more detail in the next chapter. Dieting is rarely the answer, because weight-loss diets usually entail cutting calories, and when your body doesn't get enough calories it resorts to burning muscle as well as fat. You want to preserve every bit of your muscle, because it's very hard to rebuild.

CALORIES IN VERSUS CALORIES OUT

Back when I was training for world records in both the Ironman Triathlon and the age-group fitness records at the Cooper Clinic in Dallas, Texas, my weekly mileage consisted of seventy-five miles of running, 400 miles of cycling, and five miles of swimming. One would think that I could have eaten anything I wanted without gaining weight. Well, such was not the case. Because I was then eating a lot of grains—such as oatmeal, brown rice, and whole grain bread—I found that I more than made up for the calories I burned with just a few indulgences. I was not necessarily eating "bad" foods, but I want to stress the point that it is much easier to take in lots of calories than it is to burn them off. For instance, a large muffin could easily contain 800 calories, which you would have to run about eight miles or walk sixteen miles to burn off. That is why you need to understand how diet and exercise interact.

Running a ten-minute mile for an hour burns approximately

600 calories, depending on your size and running speed. Put another way, running one mile burns 100 calories. Walking the same distance, one mile, again depending on size and speed, on average only burns 50 calories, while walking one hour only burns 150 calories. You can see, therefore, that if you want to save a lot of exercise time, you're far better off with a run. You can also see that the choices you make in the foods you eat can make a major difference in weight control. Stick to whole vegetables and fruits if you want to stay lean and low in body fat and still have all the energy you need to do all the things you want to do without getting tired.

There has also been a trend towards "super-sizing" portions both at home and in restaurants. The standard serving bowls of the past are now considered small, and dinner plates have been getting larger. A "super-sized" meal at McDonald's may contain double the calories of the standard size, and most people will eat all that's put in front of them. These factors contribute to the epidemic of obesity in this country.

THE NEW FOOD PYRAMID
OR EATING BY COLORS

You've probably heard some old adages such as "Everything in moderation" and "There's no such thing as a 'bad' food," or "There is a place for everything in a well-planned diet." This, I believe, is where most people get into trouble. The "moderation" myth clearly does not hold for arsenic, cigarettes, and animal foods. In fact, Caldwell Esselstyn, MD, flatly rejects this myth. Based on his research at the Cleveland Clinic in Ohio,[21] Esselstyn has a different message: "Moderation kills!"[22] Now, it is true that one can sometimes get away with consuming "moderate" amounts of these products for a while, but for us mature folks who do not want to settle for just "moderate" health or "moderate" rates of heart disease and cancer, I recommend staying away from all three of those products.

Another source of advice—the government-approved Food Guide Pyramid—has also not been very effective in leading us to good health. This is partly because the pyramid is based not on science, but on suggestions from the people on the decision-making panel. A majority (six out of eleven) represent the meat and dairy industries and fight very hard to keep their products in the Food Guide Pyramid. The Physicians Committee for Responsible Medicine (www.pcrm.org) in 2003 won a lawsuit against the USDA,[23] charging that these decision-makers had financial interests in the meat and dairy industry. However, it was too late to stop the existing Food Guide Pyramid from getting published. This is an example of our government leading us astray with bad information.

The best way to choose healthy foods is to choose whole plant foods in as many colors as possible. Picture bright red strawberries and cherries, vibrant oranges, bell peppers in green, yellow and red, deep green leafy greens, purple grapes, deep blue blueberries, and black blackberries. In this way, you'll get the phytonutrients described above, keep calories in line, get lots of fiber, and enjoy truly healthful eating.

WHAT ABOUT SUPPLEMENTS?

If you were to look up the Recommended Daily Allowances (RDA) for all the known nutrients, you would find that fruits and vegetables provide more than enough for each one of them, with the exception of B-12 (more on that later). I have already discussed how there is adequate protein in plant foods and that, in fact, there is a risk of getting too much. Therefore, you don't need to take protein supplements when eating plant foods, as long as you're getting enough calories. A varied diet with lots of fruits and vegetables provides more than enough of the vitamins and minerals required to be healthy.

You should be aware that you could actually be causing a problem by taking supplements, since some vitamins can be toxic when taken in large doses, and taking mega-doses of some minerals can actually interfere with the absorption of other vital minerals. There are also other problems. When, for instance, the popular press reported that tomatoes seemed protective for prostate cancer, it was thought that the carotenoid lycopene was responsible for the curative power, since this is the phytochemical that tomatoes (and other red-pigmented fruits and vegetables) have lots of. So, driven by a thirty-second media spot, men over the age of forty rushed out and bought the lycopene supplements that are now so eagerly provided by profit-driven vitamin companies. Their inductive logic was clear: "Those who consume a lot of tomatoes have less prostate cancer. Tomatoes contain a lot of lycopene. Lycopene must be what's preventing prostate cancer. Therefore, taking a lycopene supplement should prevent prostate cancer." But that logic didn't go far enough, because it wasn't at all clear that lycopene alone was responsible for the risk reduction. A University of Illinois study[24] demonstrated that pure lycopene provides far less protection than the whole tomato and that there are protective factors in the tomato beyond just the lycopene—or, more likely, that something is needed in combination with lycopene that is *not* provided by the supplements.

This raises three concerns with supplementation: (1) conclusions are often based superficially on limited research; (2) a concentrated dose of any single chemical can and often does have unintended consequences; and (3) people often try to justify taking a pill as an alternative to a healthy diet. The conclusion: Eat lots of tomatoes, tomato products, and other red-pigmented fruits and vegetables, and skip the lycopene supplements.

Another problem with supplements is that they are frequently used to treat just the symptoms—just as most modern Western medicine does—and totally ignore the *cause* of those symptoms. There are three radio talk shows about health that I regularly listen to—two national and one local. The conversation usually goes like this: "Yes, thank you for taking my call. I've just been diagnosed with IBS, irritable bowel syndrome. What should I do?" "You should take 'bowel-soothe'" or some such supplement. I have never heard the answer, "Increase your intake of fruits and vegetables." Another frequent example: "I have terrible PMS." (This usually refers to Premenstrual Syndrome, but could also mean Post Menopausal Symptoms.) The answer usually is to take "women's formula" or some such supplement. Again, I have never heard, "Clean up your diet by eating more fruits and vegetables, and get some daily, vigorous exercise." Our whole society seems to be oriented to just treating the symptoms of an unhealthy lifestyle and never getting at the *cause* of the problem. Of course, there's a lot of money to be made when you sell supplements. Furthermore, when you only treat the symptoms, you have a customer for life, because the symptoms will continue indefinitely.

You may have read that the *Journal of the American Medical Association* has recommended that "everyone" take a daily multiple vitamin pill.[25] When you look closely at what they are saying, however, it tells a very different story. Based on surveys, it was found that very few Americans eat the recommended five fruits and vegetables per day and therefore are deficient in vitamins and minerals. In fact, according to the National 5-A-Day Committee, only thirty-six percent of Americans are even *aware* that they should be consuming the recommended five servings of fruits and vegetables daily.[26] Consider, too, that those who are *not* eating the five servings a day are, by definition, replacing those foods with animal foods—with all their cholesterol, saturated fats, excess protein, etc. To expect that taking a little vitamin pill will undo all that damage is ludicrous. If, however, you're eating a well-planned vegan diet, you know that 100 percent of your diet consists of healthy, whole, plant foods and that you are getting your vitamins and minerals through "real" food and in the right amounts, B-12 excepted.

WHAT ABOUT VITAMIN B-12?

The only nutrient that most, but not all, agree might be lacking in an all-plant diet is Vitamin B-12, which is made by bacteria and stored in animal tissues. We need B-12 to synthesize red blood cells and keep our nervous system intact. Children need it to grow and develop properly. If we don't have enough, we can become anemic and destroy the nerve fibers throughout our body, including our brain. While some have tried to find B-12 in plant forms, most of the B-12 that is available for us is in foods supplemented with B-12 or in animal products. While there are a number of B-12 analogues—"look-alike" molecules that fit the receptor sites in cells—they don't do the job of the real B-12.[27]

Part of the reason for the deficiency of B-12 in our diets is that our food has become so disinfected and sanitized that there remain no traces of bacteria on the vegetables that grew in the soil. While some authorities believe that after the switch from the SAD diet to a vegan diet there is enough B-12 stored in our bodies to last several years, others strongly recommend a daily, reliable source of B-12. In any case, to be sure you are not deficient, it is safest to take some form of B-12, either in a pill or in fortified foods such as nutritional yeast with B-12.[28]

B-12 deficiency is by no means a problem associated solely with vegans. There is also some evidence that many people over fifty may be deficient in B-12.[29] The *Tufts University Health & Nutrition Letter* (June 2003) recommended that since older people may have trouble absorbing this vitamin, they should get a regular source of B-12. There was also a study that looked at two hundred frail, elderly women and found that osteoporosis occurred more often in those with low or marginal levels of B-12.[30]

We also now know that a B-12 deficiency can raise levels of homocysteine beyond normal.[31] This can cause damage to the walls of the arteries and raises your risk of heart disease, depression, and dementia.[32]

You need to know that all nutrients work in concert with each other and that by taking a large amount of one nutrient in a supplement you may be blocking the absorption of others. Too much of one may also affect how others are used in the body. Nutrients have a synergy that can never be duplicated in a pill—and, of course, many more have yet to be discovered. My advice would be to consult your doctor and have regular check-ups and blood tests to determine your B-12 levels.

WHAT ABOUT VITAMIN D?

This so-called "vitamin" is not actually a vitamin but a hormone that the body makes in response to the sun shining on the skin. It is, nevertheless, necessary, and it is thought that as we age it is more difficult to get enough of it. If you are getting daily exercise outside, you are probably getting enough Vitamin D, but people restricted to indoors or who live year-round in the northern climates should consider a Vitamin D supplement. It is a necessary component to maintaining strong bones and muscles. In one study published in the November 2003 issue of the *Journal of the American Geriatrics Society*, it was found that of almost a thousand older women (average age eighty-four), those who fell tended to have lower Vitamin D levels than those who didn't.[33]

WHAT ABOUT JUICING?

I'm often asked about the advantages and disadvantages of juicing. My own preference is to eat the whole food. After all, our jaw muscles, the mandible and maxilla (the jawbones), and even our teeth and gums need exercise. Chewing food thoroughly also gives the food a chance to be thoroughly mixed with our salivary enzymes that start the digestion process in the mouth. Juicing also robs our body of the fiber that plays such an important role in our digestive tract. There is no comparison between eating the whole food and drinking just the juice. My advice: Eat the fruit, the whole fruit, and nothing but the fruit!

EATING IN RESTAURANTS

Eating out has become such a part of our social and business lives that many cannot imagine life without restaurants and fast food outlets. While vegans don't have to give up eating out completely—and there are many restaurants that serve only vegan or vegetarian food—you do have to make some adjustments to eat healthfully. Nearly all restaurants have vegetables and fruit somewhere on the menu, and most waiters will try to accommodate you in serving what you would like. You may wish to call ahead of time to make sure they have the foods you want. You can always make a meal out of a steamed vegetable platter (my mainstay for years!) and order a bowl of strawberries and blueberries for dessert. I recommend avoiding the dressings and sauces, because most prepared foods have a myriad of unhealthy ingredients added. Stick to whole, preferably raw fruits and vegetables, and even order double servings if you must to get the quantity you need. Buffets are also a possibility with their wide range of raw fruits and vegetables—if you are good at avoiding temptation!

FOOD SAFETY

While all food should be washed and clean, the safest foods to eat are clearly plant foods. Food-borne pathogens grow in animal tissue, and since we have the same tissue we are susceptible to food poisoning from those same pathogens. It is impossible to sterilize beef in a slaughterhouse or chicken in processing plants, and inspections are inadequate. Although irradiation is effective in sterilizing food, the idea is not appealing to most of us.

Bacteria and viruses can be transferred by hands, cutting boards, and kitchen utensils. Animal foods are a source of contamination if they come in contact with plant foods, so be sure that your food is handled safely. This is difficult, if not impossible, if there are animal foods in your kitchen or the restaurant's kitchen. Eating tainted food results in 76 million cases of gastrointestinal illnesses, 325,000 hospitalizations, and 5,000 deaths every year,[34] and there have been many medical warnings to people to limit their consumption of fish due to the PCBs, toxic metals such as mercury and cadmium, and high levels of pesticides they contain.[35] Given these figures, it is very hard to avoid tainted food entirely. Nevertheless, if you follow a healthy lifestyle, you will be more likely to have a stronger immune system to fight off infection.

WATER

Although most of us don't think of water as a nutrient, it is essential that we get enough of it. Our bodies are approximately two-thirds water. Water is used in every action of every enzyme, in carrying nutrients in our bloodstream, in regulating body temperature, and more. Most people need more water than they get, although a few drink too much. If you overdo it, you get a condition called hyponatremia, where the blood has too low a concentration of electrolytes. This can be life-threatening. The easiest way, in general, to tell if you're drinking enough is to look at the color of your urine. It should be pale yellow. If it is dark, head for the water fountain. Although this test is not foolproof, it's the best we have without access to a medical laboratory. You need to know, too, that you need to drink at least nine consecutive swallows because that's the quantity it takes to trigger the pylorus, the valve at the bottom of the stomach, to empty the water into the small intestine where it is best absorbed into the bloodstream. Other than that, you can't really go by a given quantity because there are too many variables—such as your size, perspiration rate, consumption of high-water-content foods such as raw fruits and vegetables, the ambient temperature, and your activity level—to determine adequate water consumption.

THE TARAHUMARA INDIANS

The Tarahumara Indians of the Copper Canyon, Mexico are famous for their endurance running games, lasting from twenty-four to forty-eight hours. I'd read about them and decided to see for myself if this was really true or just another myth. Therefore, in February 2003, I visited them and confirmed what I'd read. They are an excellent example of the interaction between diet and exercise. They call themselves "rarauri," with "rara" meaning "runners" and "uri" meaning "steep," because of the steep canyons where they live. Copper Canyon is four or five times the size of our Grand Canyon. The Tarahumara play a game called "rarajipare" that consists of two teams of seven each. Runners flip the ball with the top of their foot as far as they can, and both teams run to capture the ball. This continues all day and throughout the night, and then through the next day and night, usually lasting up to three days and nights until only one player remains. They play by lighted torches at night and consume "tasguino," milled corn mixed with water, as their only food. By the end of the game, the men have run an average of 200 miles. The women have their version of the game as well, and they average 100 miles.

Medical tests of the Tarahumara have found that they have very low total cholesterol, averaging 125 mg/dl, and low HDLs, around 25. With their diet primarily of corn, their risk of our Western chronic degenerative diseases is extremely low, so they have no need for high HDLs. They are also formidable competitors in endurance races in the United States and will continue to be unless their exposure to our Western ways changes their diet and exercise patterns.[36]

BOTTOM LINE—WHAT WE KNOW FOR SURE

Unfortunately, nutritional information can get so complex that most people don't bother to read it or even try to understand it. Actually, you don't really have to understand the basic chemistry and physics of nutrition. What you *do* need to understand is what *is* good for you—whole plant foods—and what is *not* good for you—animal foods. It's just that simple!

CHAPTER 6

Exercise—Use It or Lose It

THE DEFINITION OF FITNESS

REGARDLESS OF AGE, fitness is something we should all strive to maximize, and it's even more important for us seniors. A fit body gives us a higher quality of life. It allows us to be independent, gives us more energy, leaves us feeling alive and vibrant and able to engage in all the activities we desire, and can help keep us free of medication because we won't have the conditions of disease and disuse we talked about in the chapter on aging.

There are four components to fitness: cardiovascular fitness, muscular fitness, flexibility, and core strength. Cardiovascular fitness means having a strong heart and circulatory system and is gained by doing regular aerobic exercise. Muscular fitness is the development of strong muscles and requires stresses or loads to be put on the muscles. Lifting weights is the most common way to develop and maintain muscular fitness. The flexibility we are born with is lost over the years from lack of use unless we make a conscious effort to keep stretching the major muscle groups and put our joints through their entire range of motion daily. Core strength, or spinal stabilization, is having abdominal and back muscles strong enough to prevent one of the most common medical complaints, lower back pain. Another common result of poor core stabilization is the potbelly. So keep those abs strong!

THE DEFINITION OF EFFECTIVE EXERCISE

Probably one of the most frequent admonitions from doctors in dealing with their sick, unfit patients is to get more exercise; and probably the most frequent excuse given is, "But doc, I just don't have the time." The second most common excuse is probably the one about getting enough exercise "chasing the grandkids" or "in my job." As mentioned earlier, you will lose muscle and bone as you age unless you have an active, effective exercise program.

Effective exercise has several criteria. A mnemonic to remember is FIT: Frequency, Intensity, and Time (or duration). First, your exercise routine has to be intensive enough to raise your heart rate, make you breathe hard, and make you sweat. Then, it has to be long enough in duration to get the body into the fat-burning mode. There's a lot of leeway here, but estimates range from twenty minutes three times a week to an hour a day. That former estimate tends to be less in favor these days, as it has not been effective for most people. If you can get people to schedule an hour a day, it's more likely that they'll have the motivation to get in at least four or five days. It's also been shown that the exercise doesn't have to be done in all one session; ten minutes three times a day has as much benefit. In one study, it was found that there was greater compliance, greater weight loss, and greater cardiovascular improvement when exercise was done in shorter bouts.[1]

AEROBIC, ANAEROBIC, ENDURANCE, AND STRENGTH EXERCISE

What kind of exercise is best? The ideal is to get several different kinds of exercise over the course of a week. In general, aerobic exercise is what most people need on a regular basis. If you get no other type, this one is crucial, because you need to have a strong heart, or cardiovascular fitness. The term "aerobic exercise" was coined by Kenneth Cooper, MD, in the 1960s when he was charged with getting new Air Force recruits into shape as quickly as possible. He found that running daily for at least twenty minutes was the most effective exercise for increasing their fitness levels.[2] Running uses the largest muscles in the body, the quadriceps (thighs), the gastrocnemius (calves), and the gluteus maximus (buttocks). Running also requires a steady flow of oxygen, and as long as the running is done at a fairly comfortable level, it is considered "aerobic." If you can talk while doing your exercise, it's aerobic. This is known as the "talk test."

Anaerobic exercise is any effort that requires breathing so hard and using so much oxygen that you cannot talk. For example, a 100-yard dash at your top speed, or lifting the greatest amount of weight you could possibly handle, would be anaerobic. In fact, lifting weights is the exercise that gets you muscular fitness.

Endurance exercise is an aerobic exercise that is continued for long distances—such as marathons and channel swims. These usually have to be built up to gradually; as the body gets stronger, you can go longer and further. The rule for increasing endurance is usually no more than ten percent per week. Otherwise, if you increase too rapidly, you risk an injury through overuse.

The most popular form of strength exercise is resistance training or weight lifting. To increase strength, you should start at a weight that is comfortable enough that you could lift it eight to ten times, feeling mild fatigue at the end. As this weight becomes easy and there is no fatigue, you can either increase the repetitions or increase the weight. Most strength trainers do a combination of both. You can do a set of ten repetitions, rest for a minute or two, and then do another set of ten. When you're able to perform three sets separated by short rests, then start increasing the weight.

Strength exercise is very individual; you are the best judge of how much to do and how quickly you progress in building strength. Nevertheless, you should remember that you need to stress the muscle beyond what it is accustomed to bear in order to challenge it to get stronger. Do about five minutes of warming up such as running in place, then devote about twenty minutes to the upper body and twenty minutes to the abdominal muscles and lower body. Rest and allow your muscles to recover for two or three days. You can do both the upper and lower body in the same day or alternate upper and lower exercises. Cool down with a few minutes of gentle stretching.

STRETCHING TO MAINTAIN FLEXIBILITY

Stretching is what maintains your flexibility and should be done when your muscles are warm, after a workout. Bend over and touch your toes to stretch your hamstrings and the backs of your thighs, as this is where most people find tightness. You can also do some side stretches and arm stretches by raising your arms as high as possible and then reaching around behind your back as far as possible. Turn your head around as if to look behind you. This is an important stretch, as many people find it difficult to drive when they can't turn their heads to back up out of a driveway or see traffic behind them. Yoga classes are an excellent way to keep you flexible.

All of the different types of exercises contribute to your fitness, so it's best to devise a schedule where you cover each of these areas at least two or three times a week. With less than that, your fitness levels start to decline. You should schedule at least one type of exercise every day, and try to stick to your schedule. Things inevitably come up to interrupt your schedule, so if you miss a day, that's okay. Try never to miss two days in a row, however, because it will be much more difficult to get back on track. You will see the benefits from doing this exercise program for the rest of your life.

Another reason to think about maintaining an effective exercise program is that if you should have an accident or need surgery, you will recover much faster if you are fit. When I was diagnosed with breast cancer, I was already a marathoner and had no idea that I would bounce back from my surgery so quickly. I even sneaked in a run early in the morning of my surgery because I wasn't sure how long it would be before I could run again. I tried to get back to my hospital bed before they knew I was gone, but I didn't make it because my surgeon just happened to be coming in the hospital door as I came running up, all sweaty. He was so shocked to see me that all he could say was, "What in the world are you doing here?" I told him I just had to get one last run in before the surgery because I wasn't sure when I'd be able to run again.

Actually, I was ready to run the day after my mastectomy, but my doctor asked me to wait a day, so I really only missed one day of running—and didn't even miss any races! My surgery was on a Wednesday and I had entered a 15K (9.4 miles) race for the following Sunday. By the wildest of coincidences, the assistant surgeon, who was also a runner, was doing the same race. When I walked up to the starting line, he did a double take and his head whipped around with an expression of shock I'll never forget.

When I was hospitalized for my second cancer surgery after the biopsy, I knew that one of the things I had to get back to as soon as possible was my daily running. When we were the surgery, I asked the surgeon how soon I'd be able to get back to running. "Oh," he mused," as soon as you feel like it." That was fantastic news because I knew that I was going to "feel like it" immediately. Or so I thought.

I need to explain that I actually had to have several surgeries. The first was that excisional biopsy I described earlier, meaning that they try to cut out the entire lump. Since it was positive for cancer and the microscopic exam showed that the surgery didn't get it all—no "clear margins," as they say—I had to go back for a modified radical mastectomy: the complete removal of the rest of the breast, fascia (the sheath-like tissue covering the underlying muscle), and the axillary (armpit) lymph nodes.

My first experience with running after surgery was after that first biopsy. As it turned out, I did feel pretty good after the biopsy and ran a 10K (kilometer) race three days afterward. After all, I figured, I had already signed up for the run and paid my money, and that was enough to get me out there. Actually, I was surprised that the run was so easy. As I crossed the finish line, however, the people standing there were pointing at me with shocked and horrified expressions on their faces! I couldn't figure out what was going on. Then I looked down to where they were pointing, and, to my own horror, saw that I had bright red *blood* all over the front of my white running singlet.

In a panic, the authorities rushed me to the medical aid station, and I blurted out that I'd just had surgery and must have torn the sutures. They quickly laid me down, grabbed the scissors to cut off my running singlet, and removed the gauze bandages. I looked down at the incision. It was just as neat and clean as it could be. I could not believe it! It was only the bandage and the clothes that were bloody. What had happened was that my sweat had soaked the dried blood that was on the bandage from the surgery itself and had turned it from the dark brown color of dried blood to the bright red of fresh blood. The sutures were intact and, in fact, were healing very nicely. The surgeons had never before seen such a quick recovery. Having an effective exercise program is a form of "prehab" so you won't need as much "rehab." And you never know when you might need it.

EXERCISE STRENGTHENS AND COUNTERACTS MUSCLE AND BONE LOSS

Our bodies carry around only what we need, whether it's muscle, bone, or even memory. If you've ever had a broken arm or leg, you'll notice that when the cast comes off after six weeks or so, the muscle around the bone has atrophied to a shocking extent. While you can see the muscle loss, you can't see the bone loss. However, it's there.

The same principle applies to everyday life. We maintain only that muscle mass and bone strength we use on a day-to-day basis. We lose what we don't use. Nevertheless, the converse is also true: We can build up what we need. When stress or loading is applied to muscle and bone, they respond by getting stronger. The only caveat is that such exercise needs to be done slowly and steadily. Too much too soon will cause injury.

You often hear that walking is the "perfect" exercise, and there is no doubt that it is a good exercise. However, it has its limitations, in that for anyone who is reasonably fit, there will be no improvement after a few weeks. Certainly, if you are very unfit or chronically overweight, walking is a good place to start. However, ultimately you need to graduate from "high school" (walking) to "college" (running). Here are some of the pros and cons of walking and running.

WALKING: ADVANTAGES AND DISADVANTAGES

Walking is probably the simplest form of exercise there is. Almost anyone can do it at any time and anywhere. It's certainly cheap, requiring only a good pair of walking shoes and street clothes. Walking also requires only the minimum fitness levels to start with. Even if you initially can only walk one block, you should be able to rapidly increase how far you walk. You will burn about fifty calories per mile. The only real disadvantage is that you will soon plateau in your fitness progress and will either need to start walking farther or faster or find some hills. Eventually, you will probably get to the point where you need to take the next step, which is running.

Some prefer the sport of racewalking to running because they feel it's much easier on their bodies. Racewalking is more than just fast walking or, as some say, power walking, because there is a technique that needs to be learned. One of the rules of race-walking is that your feet must always maintain contact with the ground. Some use racewalking as an intermediary step, either going from walking to running or from running to walking.

Some people think that walking is better for you because of its low impact, but this is incorrect if you want to keep your bones strong or even get them stronger. The word "impact" sounds negative, but impact or "striking" is necessary to stimulate the osteoblasts that build new bone.[3] Walking will not be enough to do this, because it's similar to lifting a very light weight—you can lift that light weight for an hour but it won't build a bigger bicep. To build a bigger bicep, you need a heavier weight than your muscle is used to, and only a few repetitions will be necessary. You need to overload both muscles and bones in order to stimulate them to get stronger. You can read more about this in the chapter on osteoporosis.

RUNNING: ADVANTAGES AND DISADVANTAGES

Running is probably the second simplest form of exercise, sport, and recreation there is. It is also rated by Dr. Cooper as one of the most effective and efficient forms of aerobic exercise. It's very efficient because of the number of calories burned per unit of time invested. As we saw earlier, while walking for an hour burns 150 calories, running for the same length of times burns 600 calories.[4]

Running is also a very natural human activity. After learning how to walk, children learn to run—and you know how difficult it is to keep kids from running! I remember when I was a lifeguard, my main job was not saving drowning swimmers but blowing the whistle at kids who were running on the deck. By the time kids reach adulthood, many of them haven't run for a long time. However, like riding a bicycle, we never forget how to do it.

Running has many health advantages. Aside from cross-country skiing, it is the most effective calorie-burner there is. Running builds strong leg and back muscles and strong bones, and is good for the heart and lungs. It's also a great stress reliever and an effective problem-solving technique. It can be done almost anywhere at any time, and under any circumstances. Whether you run a familiar route or explore a whole new area, running can be enjoyable and gets you out of the house. Whether you're a morning person or evening person, running can be done morning, noon, or evening—any time at all. It's especially useful if you are in a hurry and can only exercise for a short time.

It's been said that it's never too cold to run; you just may not have enough clothes on! Besides, you almost always end up sweating regardless of how cold it gets. The coldest temperature I've ever run in was in the winter in Ohio—twenty-nine degrees below zero. I didn't realize it at the time; I just went out for my usual morning run and was shocked later to find out how cold it was. With the wind chill, the temperature was apparently seventy-five degrees below.

Running is also very inexpensive, requiring only a pair of good running shoes. Go to a runner's running store to get properly fitted with shoes. The shoes need not be the most expensive ones in the store, but I would recommend staying with the more popular brands. Try several pairs on, run in place for a few minutes, and make sure they feel completely comfortable. There is nothing to "break in" for running shoes, so if something doesn't feel right, try another pair. Keep in mind that you don't need "mattresses" on your feet, either. Shoes perform the basic function of protecting your feet and are not supposed to absorb all impact—impact or striking is what builds strong bones. Your feet also are able to balance and grasp the running surface better with less padding. In terms of absorbing shock, your back has little "water beds" between each vertebra that absorb shock, and exercise helps keeps them healthy as well.

The main disadvantage associated with running is that many people believe that running is too hard on the body, that it will "wear out" the joints. A medical doctor in the 1960s even thought that women should never run because it would cause the uterus to drop! Over the last few decades, however, we have come to realize that running is actually excellent exercise. The only genuine danger is when runners do too much too soon and increase the risk of injury. Runners *do* have a higher risk of overuse injuries than walkers, so increase your distance gradually.

HOW OFTEN, HOW FAR, AND HOW TO KNOW?

How often you should exercise depends on you, but exercise can easily become a good habit. For me, a daily morning run has been an ingrained habit since 1968, or, as of this writing, thirty-seven years. Because of the very positive results I've gotten from running, I've been promoting it for almost as long. I would advocate exercising daily. Then, if something comes up and you have to skip a day, you can easily get back into the groove.

"Far" is a relative term. I remember when I first started my swim training for a triathlon. "Far" was from one end of the pool to the other. Soon "far" became thirty laps in that pool. The first time I tried an ocean swim, "far" was eight hundred meters—so "far" that I had to walk back the parallel distance along the shore because I couldn't swim any further. With consistent training, "far" became two thousand meters. Soon I was doing two-mile swims easily. My longest swim was a "Waikiki Double Roughwater," which was five miles. Now, *that,* to me, is far! Then one day, while I was training on my bike for another triathlon, a truck delivering a load of kitchen cabinets plowed into me, breaking my left leg and right hip. "Far" then became walking from my hospital bed to the bathroom and, later, a swim from one end of the pool to the other. The process began all over again.

STARTING AN EXERCISE PROGRAM

In starting any exercise program, you should first have medical clearance from your physician, because the last thing you want to do is get injured or set yourself back. On the other hand, I would suggest getting a medical clearance if you *don't* have an exercise program.

When starting a program, people have been known to get so enthusiastic about exercise that they overdo it, end up with very sore muscles, and get discouraged. There are several ways to monitor your level of effort. One way to do this is to calculate your heart rate. There are heart rate monitors you can buy that make it fun to see what exercise does to your heart, or you can use the old manual system, counting the beats at your wrist and timing them with a watch.

You need to start with your maximal heart rate. Theoretically, you're born with a maximum rate of 200 beats per minute (bpm), which decreases by one bpm per year. While not truly accurate, this does give you a ballpark estimate of your present maximal heart rate. So, if you were fifty years old, your theoretical max heart rate would be 150 (200 − 50). A good exercising heart rate would be around seventy-five percent of your maximum, so calculating seventy-five percent of 150, you would come up with 115. Remember, this is just an estimate, and there are other formulae as well. Check the chart I've included to give you a heart rate to strive for, depending on your fitness goals. You should soon develop a "feel" for the "right" level of exercise intensity for you. You want to feel that you are making a good effort but certainly not hanging on the "ragged" edge, frantically gasping for air.

Whether your goal is to increase fitness levels, burn fat, or strengthen your cardiovascular system, the key is to get your heart rate to the effective intensity. The proper intensity level can be estimated by using your age as a guide. Note that there are different recommended heart rate levels for fitness, fat burning, and cardiovascular training. To find the proper heart rate, find your age at the top of the chart, rounding off to the nearest age group. Next, find the three numbers below your age. These three numbers represent your training zone for attaining whatever goal you've chosen.

EXERCISE INTENSITY

Age

50	55	60	65	70	75	80	85	90	100

Cardiovascular

50	55	60	65	70	75	80	85	90	100
140	135	130	127	125	120	115	113	110	105

Fat burning

50	55	60	65	70	75	80	85	90	100
125	121	118	113	110	107	103	100	96	90

Fitness

50	55	60	65	70	75	80	85	90	100
110	107	105	100	95	93	90	88	85	80

These are just guidelines that you can follow to let you know if you are doing enough or, conversely, doing too much. Keep in mind that you should never feel pain, but that you may feel some discomfort as your body adapts to the exercise stresses being put on it.

If you don't want to buy a heart rate monitor or stop your exercise to check your pulse, you may want to try using the perceived exertion scale. This is a measure of how you feel on a scale from zero to ten. For example, if you are sitting on the couch doing nothing, you're a zero. If you're walking along and not much seems to be happening, you are probably around a two or three. If you're walking as if you were late to an appointment, with arms pumping, you may be around a five or six. If you're running, you may be around a seven or eight. If you're being chased by a pack of hyenas, you may be a ten. Once you have an idea of where your fitness level fits on this scale of perceived exertion, try for between five and eight. This will increase your overall fitness from any exercise you're doing, be it walking, running, cycling, swimming, etc.

Another gadget that might help motivate you and make exercise more fun is a pedometer. They are relatively inexpensive and can provide lots of motivation as you count up the miles. Check your total at the end of your exercise routine, and if it's less than 5,000, try for around 10,000 steps. Remember that every little bit helps, and that some is always better than none!

The best estimate of your aerobic training zone is between sixty and ninety percent of your maximum heart rate, and the figure will depend on your current level of fitness. Picture three levels of fitness: Level 1—Sedentary, Level 2—Walker, and Level 3—Runner. (I've picked these three levels for convenience, so that I can make generalizations and still try to cover everybody's differing level of fitness.) How far to go depends on your level of fitness. For Level 1, it may be to walk only a block. For Level 2, it may be to run two blocks, walk one block, and run two more. For Level 3, it may be adding ten percent a week to your present level. My general rule for runners is "Run till it hurts, stop till it doesn't, then run some more."

No matter what your exercise: *If you experience shortness of breath, persistent pain, or feel dizzy, nauseous or faint, stop immediately. These can be serious warning signs and should be checked out by your physician.* In general, though, the body will adapt to a new stress on it if given enough time, and will let you know how you're doing in most cases. Keep in mind that our bodies sometimes "lie" to us, telling us we can do more—or less—than we are really capable of! Stay in the perceived exertion levels of around five to eight and keep a log so that you can get an overall picture of your fitness progress.

I've included an illustration of my actual exercise log, where I use different colors for running, cycling, swimming, and weights so I can see at a glance how I'm doing in all sports. You should keep in mind that this is my record for triathlon training, so it is pretty intense, as I want to stay trained in all three sports. After I did my very first triathlon, I put the bike away for a while and then had to go through re-training for the next triathlon. Struggling to regain what I had lost, I learned one of my most important lessons: **It is easier to *stay* trained and fit than it is to *get* trained and fit.**

TRAINING LOG

What you should strive for right now is to move up one level. If you're completely sedentary, remember to check with your physician to see if you are physically able to start an exercise program. Remember, too, that if you don't exercise you are no better off than the person who can't exercise. I think of this every time I see someone in a wheelchair, although there are even wheelchair divisions in a lot of races. There are no excuses for not exercising.

WHY THE FIT BODY LOVES EXERCISE

For those of you who are already at Level 3, congratulations! Let's go for "Farther and Faster." Most people, once they attain a moderate level of fitness, hate to miss an exercise session. I've known many members of the road racing community over my thirty years of racing, and typically the goals are to graduate from 5Ks to 10Ks, from half-marathons to marathons, and some even to ultra-marathons. Now I'm seeing many runners graduating to triathlons. Fitness is fun, and sometimes it takes a race to motivate you to go a little farther and faster than you would by yourself. I'm not sure why it is, but my body loves to exercise and almost resents anything that interferes with my daily triathlon.

Yes, I did just say "my daily triathlon." My breast cancer diagnosis came after fourteen years of daily running, when I believed I was the healthiest person I knew. While I was recovering from the cancer surgery, I saw the Ironman Triathlon for the first time and decided that I *had* to do one myself. I became obsessed with the excitement, the image, and the challenge of doing a race composed of a 2.4-mile swim followed by a 112-mile bike ride and then a 26.2-mile marathon. I thought, and had been told, that I might not have much longer to live, and I figured that I'd better do it while I could, since my prognosis was not good. I'd also read that cancer cells thrived in an anaerobic environment, and this was a way to get more aerobic exercise in.

This is what my daily triathlon looks like: I do an hour on a stationary bike, a short or long run depending on what I did the day before, and top it off with a short or long swim depending on whether I did a short or long run. I've been doing triathlons this way for over twenty years. I've found that, with adding weight-lifting three days a week, I've got a fitness routine that I can stick with for life. I highly recommend that you consider this for yourself, since it's a great combination of exercise, fun, and the rewards of being really fit!

Triathlons have one major advantage: They involve three different forms of exercise—running, cycling, and swimming. These competencies serve you well when you are healthy, but they are even more important when you're not. For example, if you have an upper-body injury, you can usually bike or run. If you have a lower-body injury, you can always swim without kicking if need be. Then, too, you can always keep up your weight training with the unaffected parts of your body. You also can almost always get in a pool and do some form of upper- or lower-body exercise in the water. There are many advantages to having backup forms of exercise. Remember, too, that there are different distance triathlons. The shortest ones, for example, are a 400-meter swim, a 12-mile bike ride, and a 3.1-mile run. Almost anybody can do this—so you have *no* excuse!

WHAT ABOUT OUR KNEES?

Our knees are the largest hinged joints in the body, subjected to the greatest physical stresses, and are therefore at a high risk of injury. Most of these injuries are caused by overuse, pushing our muscles and tendons beyond their ability to cope. In sedentary people, however, the main problem is underuse, since people who don't exercise lack the muscle strength to fully support the knee joint when doing just their daily activities.

A number of studies have shown that running does not increase the risk of knee injury or arthritis.[5] Scientists at the Stanford University Medical Center monitored 450 runners and 433 non-runners, all between the ages of fifty and seventy-two, over an eight-year period, and found that runners developed only one-fifth the number of knee injuries as non-runners. Female runners did even better, with ninety percent fewer knee problems.[6] Thus, far from running being bad for knees, it is sedentary living that damages the joints. Runners also have no greater incidence of osteoarthritis than non-runners. In fact, research has shown that the knee cartilage is thicker in runners and joint spaces are wider and smoother.[7]

Damage done to joints is most often caused either by injury from twisting in sports such as football, skiing, baseball, etc. or, very commonly, bits of animal protein from cows, pigs, fowl, or fish, which the body considers a foreign protein. When these fragments get lodged in the joint capsule, they cause inflammation as the body tries to reject the foreign protein.[8] The obvious treatment is not to take a pill but to stop eating the animal protein.

The most common types of knee injury are ligament damage,

meniscus injuries, tendonitis, and bursitis. The knee has four major ligaments that are like tightly woven cables limiting the range of motion. If during soccer or skiing, for example, those ligaments get pushed beyond their limits, a sprain or tear may result. Most sprains heal on their own, although a tear may require surgery.

There are two menisci in the knee that act like rubber washers to cushion the femur (thigh bone) and absorb shock. Sudden twisting, bending, or squatting can cause a tear in a meniscus. Small tears can heal by themselves, but major tears usually require surgical repair. Tendonitis is an inflammation of a tendon, the fibrous cord that attaches a muscle to a bone. This happens most often with overuse and improves with rest, ice, gentle stretching and strengthening exercises. If the tendon gets torn in violent trauma, surgical repair is almost always necessary. Bursitis is an inflammation of the bursa, a small, fluid-filled sac located where there is pressure on the bone and tendon. This, too, is most often caused by overuse and, if irritated, causes excess fluid that is usually eventually reabsorbed. This may take a few weeks and improves with rest.

Injuries are not usually a reason to stop all exercising. If the knee injury is serious, you can always get in the water or do upper-body exercises. Signs of serious knee injury include being unable to put any weight on the knee; the presence of pain, swelling, redness, and heat; the joint locking or giving out; and failure to improve in three or four days. Otherwise, gentle exercise maintains the knee's normal range of motion, keeps the muscles from atrophying, and makes sure the synovial fluid in the joint nourishes the surrounding cartilage and tissue.

The most important thing is to ensure that you stop short of intense pain. Moderate exercisers heal sooner than those who get total rest, and I can vouch for this, as I've used this principle of "active recovery" a number of times![9]

CROSS TRAINING

I have already mentioned that there are several different types of exercise and that there are benefits to having choices such as running, biking or swimming. Weight training is very beneficial to muscles and bones, especially as we grow older.

Hiking can be an extremely enjoyable form of exercise. All you need for hiking is waterproof, properly fitting hiking shoes, lots of water, a group or partner (or a cell phone, if you're alone), and some food, if you're going on a long hike. Water-running or aqua jogging is another form of exercise that can be very useful as a supplement to running or during recovery from injury. There are over a million sites on the Internet to give you specific information on the different exercises you can do and find groups that make it more fun. For example, "hiking" has 346,000 separate URLs, with sites that cover hiking organizations and geographical locations. There are more than 18 million running sites; I recommend the "Runner's World" website (www.runnersworld.com) as well as the American Running Association website (www.americanrunning.org. Bicycling has nearly a half a million sites, and swimming, 5.3 million sites. So there is lots of information to support whichever exercise you choose.

WHICH EXERCISE TO DO
AND WHEN TO DO IT

You don't have to have a formal program to exercise, although structure helps your chances of success. Once you are aware of the need for and benefits of exercise, you'll see all kinds of opportunities to get more of it. You can stop using the car for errands and use your feet; you can carry groceries home as a form of lifting weights; you can imagine a flight of stairs as a free exercise machine just waiting for you to climb on; you can use the stairs instead of an elevator when there's a choice. When you must use an escalator, don't just get on and stop; keep walking—or even run up the steps and get there twice as fast. I've noticed that when I keep walking up an escalator or on moving sidewalks such as at airports, people around me will start to do it as well. Exercise can be contagious!

All these little exercise moments are beginning steps toward more intense and longer periods of exercise. We all need about an hour of concentrated exercise every day to be really fit. Whether you run, bike, swim, or do something else, find the exercise you'll do, and do it.

People frequently ask me when the best time is to exercise. The answer is "Whenever you'll do it"! Our bodies all have their own natural rhythms. Body temperatures vary 1.5 degrees between our low and high activity levels. We tend to want to be more active at the higher levels. We also know that some people are morning exercisers and some evening. I much prefer exercising in the morning and can easily go three to four hours before starting to realize I haven't yet eaten. As we'll see later, morning exercise helps people with sleep problems. I also know that my slowest marathons were the Boston Marathon, which started at noon, and the Moscow Marathon, which started at four P.M. I have also found that if any crises occur, they don't interfere with my run because I've usually already done it. That said, the best time to exercise is still whenever you'll do it.

From time to time, you may find that your exercise routine is disrupted—for example, by a long trip where exercise opportunities are severely curtailed. Don't expect to pick up where you left off when you return. My advice would be to drop back to about half the distance (or half the weight for lifting) and see how it feels. Then you can gradually get back to where you were over a period of two to three weeks.

One problem with defining "exercise" is that what most people mean when they say they are "active" or "get some exercise" is not enough. I believe that, generally speaking, "more is better." I don't believe that a twenty-minute walk three times a week is going to be as beneficial as an hour of daily, heart-pounding, heavy-breathing, sweaty running, biking, or swimming. While it *is* possible to overdo exercise, I know very few people at risk of that. I *do* know, however, that most people do far too little exercise. Our body was made to move, to gather all its own food and water, and to survive without the processed, refined, sorry excuse for "food" that we drive in a car to pick up at the corner supermarket or fast food outlet.

THE RIGHT DIET FOR EXERCISE

The body needs fuel to perform any of its functions. Diet is very important for exercise, because when blood sugar gets too low, you don't have the energy to do much of anything. Blood sugar—glucose—is the preferred fuel for the body, and this comes from carbohydrates. The body is not particular about what the source of the carbs is, whether they are simple or complex, but runners know that the best foods are plant foods. When we run low on blood sugar, in the parlance of runners we "hit the wall"; in the parlance of cyclists, we "bonk." It doesn't take athletes long to discover which foods are best for getting the body going again—it's fruit, whole fruit, and nothing but the fruit!

When we run out of the easily utilized carbs, however, the body does have its backup mechanisms. It will start to burn fat and protein, but this form of fuel involves a much more difficult process and will start to break down muscle. The body much prefers carbohydrates and will take a carb over anything else anytime.

After a long bout of exercise, your muscles will have used up their glycogen, and fruit, in particular, will help refuel those hungry muscles and start the recovery process. Studies show that the best time to restore the muscles' energy is within fifteen minutes of stopping.[10] This is when the muscles soak up the carbohydrates like a sponge and turn them into glycogen, getting ready for that next bout of exercise.

Earlier, I mentioned keeping a log to record your exercise sessions. Get a calendar that has a month at a glance and plan your schedule for the coming month. For example, my calendar notes that I spend an hour on the bike and an hour running each day. I do a swim workout on Monday, Wednesday, and Friday, and lift weights on Tuesday, Thursday, and Saturday, frequently with a race on Sunday. I'm especially lucky living in Hawaii and having access to a pool and the ocean, so I wind up swimming just about every day. After each session, I have added comments such as "Extra long bike" or "Ran the hills hard." This way I can tell if I need to do a shorter bike the next day or an easy run after the hill work.

If you're a beginner, you shouldn't be intimidated by what I have written above. I was once somebody who did little or no exercise. You should know that anybody can build up strength and fitness levels from any starting point by consistent exercise. You can also see the progress you're making by adding to your log your time, the distance you covered, and comments on how you felt.

BOTTOM LINE—WHAT WE KNOW FOR SURE

Exercise has to be a priority in your life. It is tied to our survival and our quality of life. We fail rapidly when confined to bed, because muscles and bone start to atrophy; our breathing slows, leaving us vulnerable to pneumonia; our heart loses its ability to pump blood efficiently; digestion slows; constipation occurs; and much more. Although exercise consumes more energy, it paradoxically gives us more energy. It keeps our joints mobile, helps us deal with psychological stress, and helps us sleep better. You should look for ways to vary exercise routines so that if you must travel or for some reason can't do your normal exercise, you are ready with alternatives. Remember, start at your own level, whatever that is. You don't have to be able to run a marathon next week or next month, but you should set a goal of moving up to the next level. You'll be pleased and excited to see the progress your body is capable of.

CHAPTER 7

REVERSING CARDIOVASCULAR DISEASE—HEART DISEASE AND STROKE

WHY HEART DISEASE IS WELL KNOWN, PREVENTABLE, AND REVERSIBLE

THERE ARE MORE than 1.5 million heart attacks in this country every year, and more than 500,000 of them are fatal.[1] Even scarier is the fact there are more than three million silent heart attacks, in which people aren't even aware of them or else assume that they are suffering from indigestion or another problem.[2] Heart attacks are by far the most common cause of death in this and all the other countries where people eat the way we do.

In the early 1950s, researchers looked around the world to see if they could figure out why some countries had low rates of heart disease and others high. They found some major differences.

88

We've already mentioned that during the Korean War researchers looked at the arteries of the young men who were killed in combat. What they found was that Korean men had arteries with virtually no plaque and that American men had a lot. When children are fed an animal-based diet, this process of plaque formation begins as early as two years of age.

It has been more than forty years since American scientist Ancel Keys discovered the connection between diet and heart disease. The Framingham Study found that anyone with total cholesterol below 150 mg/dl was virtually immune to a heart attack.[3] The Seven Countries Study showed the same thing—that in parts of China and Africa, heart disease was nonexistent.[4]

For years, the standard level for total cholesterol was set at 300 mg/dl, based on averages of measurement of the population. Because it was the average, it was considered "normal." But when it was shown that people with cholesterol lower than 150 did not get heart attacks, the standard was lowered to 200, a reading that many people, surprisingly, still believe to be low enough. When you consider, however, that thirty-five percent of heart attacks occur in people with total cholesterols of between 150 and 185, it becomes clear that the standard rate needs to be lowered once again. This also explains why you'll hear people denigrate the importance of cholesterol readings by saying that people with "normal" cholesterols still get heart attacks. "Normal" in this country is around 220, but, as we have seen, "normal" in China is 120, and "normal" among the Tarahumara Indians of Northern Mexico is 125.

It should be noted that there is a recent trend to break down the total cholesterol into HDL and LDL, and it is very important to have a high HDL and low LDL when your total cholesterol is above 150. However, your goal should be to get the total down below 150, where you can put yourself in that group of those "virtually immune" to a heart attack, and where your total cholesterol is as low as that of the Tarahumara runners.

Besides cholesterol readings, I've mentioned other blood tests for heart disease: C-reactive protein, lipoprotein (a), and homocysteine. An elevated level of inflammation can increase your risk of a heart attack. Elevated homocysteine levels, for example, can damage the cells that line artery walls and stimulate overgrowth of the smooth muscle cells and fibrous tissue. Homocysteine also releases elastase, a substance that destroys the flexibility of the artery. This results in thickened, tough, hardened artery walls lined with clot-filled deposits. The plaque itself or a migrating clot can block an artery, cutting off the blood flow to the heart or the brain and triggering a heart attack or stroke. Studies show some vegans with low B-12 levels have high homocysteine levels, and at least 200 studies have confirmed that elevated homocysteine is a major risk factor for heart disease and stroke.[5] Just as with high cholesterol readings, a healthy low-fat vegan diet with adequate B-12 usually lowers these readings to a healthful range.

THE MEDITERRANEAN DIET
AND THE ASIAN DIET

The Mediterranean Diet is without question better than the Standard American Diet (SAD). Three studies conducted in Greece, Italy, and Spain in 2003 found that a diet with lots of vegetables, fruit, and grains lowered the risk of dying from all causes.[6] The Italian study included survivors of recent heart attacks. Unfortunately, while these Mediterranean diets are better than many diets, they don't go far enough, because they still include fish, cheese, and refined oils. As the evidence of the following three studies suggests, the results for the Italian survivors would have been even better if they had avoided all animal foods and refined, processed foods.

The Asian Diet is even better in terms of lowering the risk of heart disease and many other diseases. Most Asians cannot tolerate dairy products, so that one fact alone gives the Asian Diet an advantage over the Mediterranean Diet. Asians also tend to use much less oil in their cooking. The best research in this area has been done by T. Colin Campbell, PhD, of Cornell University, in the comprehensive and long-term China Diet Study.[7] Dr. Campbell found that the lower the fat, the healthier the people— with no lower limit. He found the healthiest people ate diets as low in fat as five percent. Not surprisingly, these were the poorest people, who tended to live in the most rural areas where their access to animal foods was the most restricted. Dr. Campbell now follows a vegan diet and runs daily.

THE ORNISH AND ESSELSTYN RESEARCH

Dean Ornish, MD, has conducted a significant amount of research on heart disease and its reversal. He was not the first doctor to do this, but he has gotten the most publicity with the publication of his book *Reversing Heart Disease*, and his study results were published in a major medical journal.[8]

Ornish took a number of people with documented heart disease and put them on a low-fat vegetarian diet. To make sure his program would give his patients their best chance of success, he added exercise, group support, and stress reduction through meditation. After a year, angiograms showed a significant reversal in the narrowing of the patients' coronary arteries and a lessening of the symptoms of their condition. Unfortunately, this program has not been as widely adopted as it should have been, mainly because the mainstream media has dismissed it as somehow "cultish" and its regimen "too hard to follow."

Caldwell Esselstyn, another MD researching heart disease reversal, has, in the longest-running study to date, achieved better results even faster using diet combined with statins.[9] Esselstyn is one of America's most esteemed cardiologists. He hangs his shingle at the Cleveland Clinic, which *U.S. News and World Report* has recognized for a number of years as the finest heart treatment center in the United States, and America's third best hospital after Johns Hopkins and the Mayo Clinic. Esselstyn states:

> The Cleveland Clinic has been the top ranked heart clinic for eight years in a row. Top ranked not in preventing heart disease, but simply in ripping it out once you get it. How do we keep those wheels churning? How do we keep the tables busy? Well, we have a McDonald's on the first floor! And we then treat people on the second floor.[10]

The diet in Esselstyn's study is vegan—with no animal products or oil whatsoever. (Ornish's diet allows some skim milk and egg whites.) Dr. Esselstyn's patients kept their total calories from fat under ten percent. His goal was to get their total serum cholesterol below 150 and their LDL below eighty.

By following a strict, low-fat vegan diet, most people see *significant* reductions in their cholesterol levels in less than two to three weeks. Such losses are relative, however. At a recent talk I attended, Dr. Esselstyn gave the example of a colleague of his, a forty-four-year-old physician who had a total cholesterol of 156 and who *still* had a heart attack. Being aware of Dr. Esselstyn's study, the doctor—after discovering that his anterior descending coronary artery was blocked—went on this stricter version of the program and with absolutely no medication got his cholesterol down to eighty-nine! We saw slides of his heart before the diet, with a severe blockage, and after the diet, where the descending coronary artery looked completely normal and wide open. He, too, is now a believer.

Many doctors speak in terms of "risk factors" when assessing an individual's chances of getting heart disease. At a California conference, Dr. Esselstyn commented: "I hate risk factors. We're all walking toward a cliff and risk factors only indicate how quickly you're walking. Wouldn't it be easier to just say, 'Here's the diet you can eat where you will never, ever, have this disease'?"[11]

As part of his lectures, Dr. Esselstyn relates an example of how a whole nation changed its diet: "During World War II, when Norway was occupied, they took away livestock and dairy and the populations were subsisting on plant foods. . . . [D]eaths from stroke and coronary heart disease plummeted for the duration of the war, during times of greatest stress and duress." While we know that just restricting calories can help in controlling heart disease, we also know that meat and dairy are major sources of saturated fat and cholesterol. Of course, the deaths went back to previous high levels when old eating habits were resumed after the war.

Since 1985, Caldwell Esselstyn has been the lead researcher in a study that has *proven* that heart disease can be reversed by eating a low fat, plant-based diet. In August 1999, in the *American Journal of Cardiology,* Esselstyn published his groundbreaking work proving that patients who have experienced strokes or episodes of advanced coronary artery disease can abolish or reverse disease progression by eating a low-fat, vegan diet. A stroke, after all, is really just a "heart attack" of the brain. Esselstyn described "little white spots" in patient's MRIs of the brain as evidence of tiny strokes, resulting in loss of cognition and mental function.[12]

As a young medical student in 1956, Esselstyn won an Olympic Gold Medal in Melbourne, Australia as a member of America's rowing team. He is now in his sixth decade of practice and has not slowed down. In between seeing patients, Dr. Esselstyn's passion is to spread the word that heart disease can be reversed. When asked whether it was okay to eat an occasional steak or slice of pizza, Esselstyn replied: "Now we know that a single fatty meal compromises coronary flow. This is true even in young people. Arteries are crying for oxygen; you can see it with a scan five minutes later; 120 minutes later, the effects are still obvious." Dr. Esselstyn will not take patients unless they agree to strike from their vocabulary the phrase, "Sweetheart, just this little bit can't hurt," because he knows that it can! One of the titles of a slide he uses in presentations proclaims, "Moderation Kills!"

SCAFF'S PATIENT MARATHONERS

For a number of years after the running boom of the 1970s started, it was thought that if you could run a marathon you would be forever exempt from a heart attack. In fact, Thomas Bassler, MD, a pathologist and medical examiner for the County of Los Angeles, made the claim that he guaranteed no marathoner would ever die of a heart attack.[13] It was true that runners developed a healthy blood supply to the heart, had a lower body fat percentage, and were in general much healthier than the average population. They also thought they could eat anything they wanted as long as they kept on running. Unfortunately, that turned out not to be true.

The myth of indestructibility lasted until the running guru Jim Fixx, author of *The Complete Book of Running*, died of a heart attack in 1983 while he was running.[14] It turned out that he, too, had blocked coronary arteries. The initial reaction of the public and the press was to discount the health benefits of running and to assume that running was indeed dangerous. In fact, I remember a number of people at that time saying to me, "See? That's proof that running is not good for you!" No one at the time looked at Fixx's diet and the resulting high cholesterol level of 271, because if they had it would have been obvious that it was not the running that killed him but his diet.

A cardiologist, Jack Scaff, also a runner, decided that the health benefits of exercise were so great that it would probably help people who had already had a heart attack but were lucky enough to have survived it. Up to that time, the treatment following a heart attack was weeks of complete bed rest. Scaff tried a radical approach—that of getting patients, literally, up and running. You can imagine the shock of other cardiologists; they thought that Scaff was going to kill his patients. Instead, they got stronger. To this day, Jack Scaff is still running his marathon clinics and has finally gotten the professional recognition that he deserved. He has proven that exercise is good for hearts, both sick and well.[15] Just think how much better off those hearts would be if they were fed a good diet in addition to good exercise!

YOUR OWN CORONARY BYPASS SURGERY

When you start an exercise program, the working muscles suddenly demand more oxygen. If the exercise continues, they demand more fuel (glycogen), which is initially stored in the muscles and liver. When that gets used up, then the fuel comes from glucose in the blood. When that, too, gets used up, we come to an abrupt halt until we get refueled by eating, preferably "good" carbs, fruits and vegetables. Part of the process of adapting to an increasing demand on muscles involves the body laying down new blood vessels to carry more blood—that is, more oxygen and glycogen. It has been noted that people who have blocked coronary arteries but are heavy exercisers create their own bypass in the form of new blood vessels.[16] Exercise can be a lifesaver.

STRESS

As stated in an earlier chapter, heart attacks were once thought to be caused by stress. While stress may play a role in heart disease, it is not the primary cause. One only has to look around the world and see where life is lived under extreme stress, where you would expect to see an increase in the incidence of heart attacks. As mentioned earlier, during World War II people in Norway, England, and Finland endured extreme hardships. Food was severely limited; meat, milk and butter were rationed when, or if, available, and many lived through the horrors of nightly bombing raids and losing their homes. Amazingly, the rate of heart attacks went down, not up. After the war ended, however, when meat, milk and butter became available again, the rate of heart attacks went back up to pre-war levels. So much for stress leading to heart attacks.

BOTTOM LINE—WHAT WE KNOW FOR SURE

It is clear to most scientists and medical researchers that cardiovascular and heart disease is a symptom of eating a rich, animal-based diet, and that even when well established in a patient, most of the damage can be reversed by a change to a low-fat vegan diet and daily, vigorous exercise. It is also clear that strokes are symptoms of eating that same diet with lack of exercise, and that strokes could be avoided by eating a vegan diet and exercising as well.

CHAPTER 8

STOP CANCER IN ITS TRACKS

WHY CANCER ISN'T CURABLE

THE FIRST THING you need to know about cancer is that it is, in part, a failure of the immune system. Logically, therefore, we should be doing all we can to keep our immune systems strong. A low-fat vegan diet and regular, effective exercise have both been shown to boost the immune system. In the United States, we have concentrated on trying to cure cancer rather than trying to prevent it from happening in the first place. Cancer appears in hundreds of different ways, so it is very unlikely that there will ever be a single cure for a disease that is so multifaceted.

The second thing you need to know about cancer is that there are cancer "initiators" and "promoters." For example, a mutation in a breast cell can initiate a cancer, but without a promoter such as estrogen, it will not grow. Radiation from the sun or x-rays can also be an initiator, but if the diet is high in antioxidants, the immune system will zap that cell before it has a chance to spread. Correlational studies seem to indicate that a diet high in fat and animal protein is a promoter. Since we can't control many of the initiators of cancer, it is crucial that we keep our immune systems strong, because that's the only way we can prevent or control cancer. Although pharmaceutical companies are searching for "magic bullets" to "cure" cancer, it is far better to prevent it by a healthy lifestyle.

As a cancer patient myself, I have noted that for the past twenty-two years, newspapers and magazines have regularly been reporting "breakthroughs" in cancer treatments, but the sad fact is that survival times have not been lengthened in the most common cancers—lung and colon cancer in both men and women, and breast cancer in women and prostate cancer in men. According to the National Cancer Institute (2000), chemotherapy's overall success rate is a mere 5.8 percent,[1] although in some cancers, such as testicular cancer, chemotherapy can be very effective.

It is a fact, however, that by the time most cancers are detected by palpable lumps, x-ray, scans, blood tests, etc., the tumor has been shedding cancer cells for years. With a few exceptions such as *in situ* or locally invasive cancers, this is the nature of cancer and makes the difference between a malignant (cancerous) and benign (non-shedding) tumor. Once these rogue cells break away from the primary tumor, they are transported through the circulatory system to other parts of the body, where they set up new tumors. It is almost impossible to detect the new colonies until they, too, are large enough to be picked up by the usual diagnostic tests.

EARLY DETECTION

Early detection as promoted by well-meaning health agencies and medical professionals is really a myth for the reasons stated above. It is impossible with present-day diagnostic equipment to detect a single cancer cell by itself. The smallest palpable lump is about the size of a grain of rice and already contains millions of cancer cells. Mammograms can pick up smaller tumors but, again, there are already millions of cancer cells in the smallest possible tumor visible in any x-ray. In my own case, the tumor was the size of a golf ball and yet was not picked up on my mammogram, and I was told that mammograms miss about thirty percent of cases of breast cancer. Blood tests have the same disadvantage.

Another important thing to remember is that improved diagnostic methods simply enable the patient to find out about her disease sooner. Assume the first cell turns cancerous in 1990 and becomes palpable in 2000. Assume also that surgery, chemotherapy, and radiation fail to halt the spread of the disease and the patient dies in 2003. In this scenario, "improved mammography" discovers the tumor in 1997 instead of 2000 and the patient, instead of surviving, say, three years after diagnosis, survives six. It is said that, if you don't have a recurrence for five years, you're considered "cured." However, in our hypothetical case, the patient died in the sixth year after diagnosis. What appears to the uninitiated to be a lengthened survival time is a fiction caused by earlier diagnosis, which only *artificially* lengthens "survival" time. The natural course of the disease, in most cases, is unfortunately still the same. The statistical findings that five-year survival rates are increasing is also illusory. Let us say that twenty years ago, a tumor had to be one centimeter in size before it could be picked up on a mammogram. The prognosis for tumors that size and type was, let us say, four years of survival. Today, assume that same tumor can be picked up two years earlier, so the patient is still alive five years later. It just *appears* as if the survival time was lengthened and the patient thus is counted as a "cure"—even though he or she may die the day after the five-year mark.

There are other cancers with dismal survival rates. Lung can-

cer, for example, has a five-year survival rate of less than ten percent, meaning that fewer than one out of ten patients are alive five
years after their diagnosis. The Surgeon General's Report in 1979
reported that little significant progress in the diagnosis or treatment of lung cancer had been made in the previous fifteen years.[2]
All that has changed since then is that the mortality rate of lung
cancer in women surpassed that of breast cancer in 1987, clearly
reflecting increased smoking among females.[3]

One of the most common types of cancer has been linked to
a low-fiber diet and constipation. Constipation is the stated cause
of 2.5 million visits to the doctor and 100,000 hospitalizations in
this country every year.[4] People are sometimes told, just as I was,
that it may be normal to have only one to two bowel movements
a week. This just is not so. In a diet rich in fruits and vegetables,
you are almost guaranteed at *least* one easy-to-pass, very bulky
stool per day. Besides lowering your risk of colon cancer, regular
bowel movements will also lower your risk of hemorrhoids,
appendicitis, diverticulitis, and what some doctors claim is a system that is toxic.

SCREENING TESTS FOR CANCER

Everyone should be aware of what's going on in their bodies and
have regular check-ups. Women *and men* should examine their
breasts once a month (men can get breast cancer, too). Women
should have an annual Pap smear (unless you have had a hysterectomy or three negative tests in a row). Both men and women
should have a simple fecal occult blood test each year, and a
colonoscopy every ten years after age fifty. Men over fifty should
have a digital rectal exam along with the PSA blood test if recommended by the doctor, an annual examination of the skin from
head to toe for any suspicious moles or other growths, and any
other screening tests that seem warranted.

The American Cancer Society tells us that 1.3 million Americans will be diagnosed with cancer this year and that 565,000 of them will die of the disease.[5] You should also be aware that in the countries that don't eat the way we do, the cancer rate is significantly lower. In fact, in some developing countries, doctors will tell you they rarely ever see a case of breast cancer. Of course, this doesn't conclusively *prove* anything, but where would you place your bets? In general, therefore, if you have been following a low-fat vegan diet and getting daily vigorous exercise for a number of years, your risk of getting cancer is significantly lower. As I know personally, prevention of cancer is a far better alternative to treatment.

CHEMOTHERAPY AND RADIATION

For chemotherapy and radiation to kill all the cancer cells, the doses have to be so high that they kill, or nearly kill, the patient. These treatments can cause irreversible damage to the patient's immune system. Our immune system keeps us alive; without it, we are prey to every bug that comes along.

What confuses a lot of people is how cancer kills. Right after my diagnosis, a few people told me, "Well, you're lucky it's just a breast." What people don't realize is that it's not necessarily the primary, or first, tumor that is fatal—particularly in breast, colon, and prostate cancers. It is the metastasis, or spread, of these cells that break away and set up housekeeping in the liver, lungs, bones, and brain. *That* is what kills the patient. We can all survive the loss of a breast, or prostate if male, or live without a few feet of intestine. However, we *cannot* survive the loss of the crucial, life-giving functions of the liver, lungs, bones, and brain. Because these four sites are so rich in their blood supply, tumor cells find an environment that enables them to continue their uncontrolled, erratic growth, in a manner so wild that they strangle the host. Those cells can hide anywhere in the body, and research has shown that they can survive, despite advances in detection and treatment, for up to fifty years.[6]

Tracking down "cancerous cells" is extremely difficult, and destroying them with chemicals and radiation is not only difficult but also extremely hazardous to our normal cells. That is why chemotherapy causes nausea, vomiting, and hair loss. The normal cells most vulnerable to these weapons are the fastest-growing cells—in this case, the lining of our gastrointestinal system and hair. If chemotherapy is not powerful enough to cause those side effects, it's not likely to stop the cancer cells, either.

Another indication that surgery, chemotherapy and radiation are largely ineffective is that when women are diagnosed with breast cancer, they are usually told of the treatment options and allowed to decide what they want. This is because *none* of these options is clearly the "best" or offers a high cure rate. I don't know of any other disease you can present to a doctor and be met with an offering of options and asked to choose. If surgery *or* chemo *or* radiation really worked, you could be sure that the doctor would strongly encourage you to do the one treatment that worked and probably not even mention less effective options.

Because oncologists, or cancer specialists, are seeing so little change in the longevity of their patients with the most common kinds of cancer, a few are starting to emphasize prevention. Through epidemiological (population) studies, it is very clear that individual countries have their own patterns of frequency of the different kinds of cancers. When many of these frequencies are correlated with dietary differences, a telling pattern emerges. There was a study published in the journal of the *National Cancer Institute* in January 6, 1993 that showed that breast cancer patients who followed a low-fat diet had far fewer "treatment failures" than those who continued to eat the diet they had been following when they were diagnosed with the disease.[7] Unfortunately, I know of no large studies done where women with breast cancer were put on a low-fat vegan diet and followed for a number of years. I do know, however, that the vegan diet worked for me.

FISH AND CANCER

Some studies conducted on animals have claimed that fish and their omega 3 "good fats" have a protective effect against the risk of breast cancer, but the evidence from human population studies is limited. Researchers have also looked at the association between total fish intake and the effect of fat content and the preparation method of the fish in relation to the rate of breast cancer among postmenopausal women. They have investigated the effect of fish intake with respect to estrogen receptors in breast cancer. When they compared individuals and groups of women (case-control and cohort studies), they have rarely shown significant associations between high fish intake and low breast cancer incidence.

A total of 23,693 postmenopausal women were studied for their fish consumption and followed with a detailed questionnaire. During the five-year period that they were followed, 424 of the women were diagnosed with breast cancer. The results of this Diet Cancer and Health Study were published in the November 2003 *Journal of Nutrition*.[8] Those eating the *most* fish had a fifty percent greater risk of developing breast cancer. The researchers estimate that women may raise their breast cancer risk thirteen percent for every twenty-five grams (a quarter of a serving) of fish they eat every day. This increased breast cancer risk from fish consumption held strong even after controlling for other risk factors, such as alcohol, obesity, hormone use, etc.

MYTHS ABOUT CANCER

The most common myth about cancer is the five-year myth that we discussed earlier—a myth that lies behind some of the "miracle breakthroughs" that have been claimed. C. Barber Mueller did a follow-up study of women with breast cancer, utilizing data collected for nineteen years by the Syracuse, NY Upstate Medical Center Cancer Registry on 3,558 women, and found that twenty years after diagnosis, eighty percent of them were dead. Eighty-eight percent of those deaths were due to active breast cancer, and, regardless of the cause of death, those who had died still had active breast cancer up to twenty years after the initial diagnosis.[9] Since cancer cells can remain viable *in vitro* (living tissue in a test tube) for up to fifty years, it is critical that we all keep our immune system operating at the highest level possible.

Another myth states that cancer always spreads from tumor to lymph nodes to bloodstream to distant sites. Cancer actually spreads simultaneously via the bloodstream and the lymph nodes throughout the body to the lungs, liver, bones, and brain.[10] Another problem with breast cancer is that spread to the axillary (underarm) lymph nodes is often used as an indicator of how far the cancer has reached. This fails to take into account the possibility of a tumor in the inside (medial) half of the breast, which would drain to the center of the chest and the lymph nodes behind the collar bone, and not to the axillary nodes. These medial (inside half) lymph nodes are not used in staging (the process of determining the cancer's spread) because they are too difficult to reach to biopsy (in order to gain access to the medial lymph nodes, it would be necessary to cut through the collar bone and rib cage, major surgery that is not done because of the trauma to the patient and the former belief that the easily accessible axillary nodes are sufficient to stage the disease).

Radiating the breast or most other sites of cancer is rarely effective, because by the time of diagnosis it is too late. As we have seen, by the time a tumor is clinically detectable, the cancer cells have usually already worked their way into the bloodstream and set up housekeeping in other areas of the body.

WHY CANCER IS RARE IN SOME COUNTRIES

When one looks at the rates of cancer of countries all over the world, a telling pattern emerges: There is an almost perfect correlation between animal products in the diet and cancer rates. T. Colin Campbell has pointed out that animal protein seems to be the most critical factor—and this includes milk protein:[11]

> [It] is not that protein independently accounts for the pro-cancer effect (that's the reasoning of reductionist scientists) of animal or plant based foods; rather it is the constellation of factors that accompany proteins in animal and plant based foods and the highly integrative network of cellular reactions associated with the nutrient components of these foods that give the most compelling evidence. . . . It is time that this view of health become mainstream and to figure out ways that this might happen![12]

There is also a major problem with the published studies on dietary fat and breast cancer. Since animal foods are high in both fat and protein, the significant action to take is to eliminate the animal foods.[13] There have been some studies, such as the Harvard Nurses Study, that showed no correlation between the amount of fat in the diet and breast cancer rates. The fallacy here is that these studies had as the "low" a fat level of thirty percent, which is not really low at all. The study we need will probably never be conducted, because it will be hard to find a large group of Western women eating a diet in which only from five to fifteen percent of calories come from fat. Plant foods are in general low in protein and fat (as long as you don't add oil), and therefore are probably responsible for the low cancer rates in those countries too poor to afford much in the way of animal products.

This is why so many researchers are convinced that breast, colon, and prostate cancers are related to diet. According to the findings of K. Carroll, a researcher who first published his findings in 1975, there was a nearly perfect correlation between frequency of deaths from breast cancer and percentage of dietary fat.[14] A study published by A. Lowenfels in 1977 showed that breast and colon cancer have risen together in fifty-six countries of the world.[15] It is amazing that we have had this information buried in journals for all these years, and yet people are still killing themselves with their knives and forks!

When you look at the similarity in the rise and fall of cancer rates and the consumption of animal foods, it is striking that nearly all of the variance can be explained. In other words, there is very little "room" left for other variables such as genetics, stress, and other environmental factors. So, while we cannot do the living experiments we would need to "prove" this theory, we can take advantage of this natural experiment provided us if we are smart enough to look at the data before us. For example, the few countries that have a greater fat intake than we in the US do—the Netherlands, Denmark, and New Zealand—also have greater death rates from breast cancer.[16]

As early as 1963, Ernst Wynder, MD, president and founder of the American Health Foundation, noted that Japanese women with breast cancer survived much longer than American breast cancer patients. This has nothing to do with genes, because women of Japanese ancestry living in the US *and consuming the SAD diet* had the same survival rates as the American breast cancer patients.[17] Although this doesn't actually *prove* beyond any doubt that diet is the major factor, there are enough other supporting studies that I think it is clear that diet is exceedingly relevant as a factor.

CAN EXERCISE LOWER CANCER RISK?

In case you need another reason to exercise, low-fat bodies have a much lower incidence of cancer. "Nine different, recently published studies have suggested that regular exercise might reduce the risk of cancer," says Randy Eichner, MD, a hematologist at the University of Oklahoma Health Science Center in Oklahoma City.[18] These studies showed that inactive women had about twice the risk of breast cancer and almost three times the rate of cancer of the ovaries, uterus, cervix, and vagina. Additionally, active women had about half the rate of lymphoma, leukemia, myeloma, Hodgkin's disease, and cancer of the thyroid. There were also much lower rates of incidence of other, less frequent types of cancer.

FIBER IN BREAST, PROSTATE, AND COLON CANCER

One of the reasons why a low-fat vegan diet is protective in breast and colon cancer is that this diet is highest in fiber. Fiber acts like a sponge to mop up hormones, cholesterol, and other substances that arrive in the colon in the normal digestive processes. The liver also cleans up the blood and dumps these substances into the colon for excretion in the feces. Because the people consuming the SAD diet usually get little or no fiber, however, hormones and cholesterol get re-absorbed through the intestinal wall and increase these levels in the body. With higher levels of hormones, cell division in the breasts and prostate is excessively stimulated, increasing the risk of breast and prostate cancer. These waste products are intended to move quickly through the colon, but with low-fiber diets, they sit there for longer periods of time, exposing the walls of the intestines to carcinogens and thus increasing your risk of colon cancer. Transit times—the time of eating to excretion—should be twelve to twenty-four hours; however, in this country it tends to be thirty-six to forty-eight hours or more.[19] This is why colon cancer is one of the most common cancers in both men and women. There may be other factors involved, but it stands to reason that food has the most intimate contact with the walls of the colon. Even if carcinogens are consumed with food, compared to a slower-moving, low-fiber diet, a high-fiber diet moves things along and limits the exposure.

Another factor to consider in breast cancer is the dominance of the hormone estrogen. With a diet high in fat and rich in animal foods, estrogen levels tend to run much higher in both men and women. Changing to a low-fat vegan diet will help normalize the estrogen levels. For women who still have high estrogen levels—that is, estrogen dominance—adding natural progesterone will counteract the carcinogenic effects of estrogen. The best evidence of this comes from a recent study of women previously diagnosed with breast cancer who wanted to have another baby.[20] Up until recently they were told not to risk it. A number of women who got pregnant anyway were followed to see if their cancer recurred. The incidence of disease recurrence was twenty-three percent for women who experienced a pregnancy and fifty-four percent for women who did not. The best guess as to why this is the case is that the women who got pregnant produced large amounts of progesterone during the pregnancy, which kept the cancer at bay.

In another study, a group of women who had all been found to have suspicious lumps in their breasts were scheduled for a biopsy.[21] Half of the women while waiting for the biopsy were randomly chosen to receive progesterone cream to rub on their bodies, and the other half were given a placebo cream with no active substances. After a pathologist examined the biopsied tissues, it was found that the women who had the active progesterone cream had a much lower incidence of abnormal cell growths.

Every few years, the hypothesis that antiperspirants and deodorants may be the cause of breast cancer surfaces.[22] What is noted is that breast cancer rates are higher in women who use these products and lower in women who don't. What the hypothesis ignores is difference in diet and the fact that these products are used by women in industrialized countries, who are more likely to be eating the SAD diet, and that women in the developing world are not only less likely to eat as much meat but are also less likely to rub white stuff under their arms.

Given that it is the breakdown of flesh that produces unpleasant odors in our breath, perspiration, intestinal gas, stool, and (believe it or not) the ejaculate and vaginal secretions, it's reasonable to suggest that eating meat makes you smell bad.

WHY BEING FIT IS NOT ENOUGH

While being fit is extremely important, you can still have heart disease and cancer irrespective of your fitness levels. I am living proof of that, having been a marathoner and a daily runner for fourteen years when I was diagnosed with breast cancer and high cholesterol. It was only at that point that I learned that diet plays a major role in most cancers, especially breast, ovarian, and prostate cancer. As we have seen, colon cancer is highly correlated with the typical Western, low-fiber diet. My favorite story concerns Sir Denis Burkett, an English doctor who went to Africa and was amazed to discover that the typical African's stool was much greater in quantity than that of Burkett's countrymen. It was this revelation that led to his conclusion that fiber plays an extremely important role in maintaining good health.[23]

BOTTOM LINE—WHAT WE KNOW FOR SURE

Since cancer is mainly a failure of the immune system, it is only logical that we do all we can to maintain and even improve its function. We know that there are substances in both meat and dairy products that tend to promote cancer, and that there are phytonutrients and antioxidants in plant foods that fight cancer. The best way to reduce your risk of all cancers is to eat a low-fat, whole-food vegan diet and get daily, vigorous exercise.

CHAPTER 9

Is Type 2 Diabetes Reversible?

ARE YOU OVER forty? Are you overweight? Do you not exercise? Are you eating the SAD diet? For each "yes" answer, your risk for Type 2 diabetes goes up a notch. However, you can modify all but the first risk factor very easily—and that first risk factor is diminishing in significance as even children who meet the other three criteria are developing the disease. According to Tedd Mitchell, MD, of the Cooper Clinic in Dallas, Texas, from 1990 to 2000 the number of adults with diabetes rose by a striking forty-nine percent, affecting people from all backgrounds. Epidemiologists predict that by 2025 the incidence will double.[1] Diabetes, however, is another one of the diseases that may be prevented and reversed by following the diet and exercise plan in this book.

"DO YOU HAVE TYPE 2 DIABETES?"

This is how an advertisement in this morning's paper starts out. Then it goes on:

If you are between 18 and 70 years old, not on insulin, but you are on Glucophage or metformin, you may be eligible to participate in a nationwide clinical study and gain access to a research treatment that is otherwise unavailable. You'll get free drugs, glucose (blood sugar) testing supplies, medical care, and diabetic and nutritional counseling.

But you will *never* see an ad that says, "If you have Type 2 diabetes, here's how you can reverse it. Go on a low-fat vegan diet and start exercising daily!" The reason for this is the same for many medical conditions: There is a *lot* of money to be made on the former advertisement and none on the latter!

Additionally, you should know that the purpose of Glucophage and metformin is to try to sensitize the receptor sites to insulin, and that exercise will do the same thing—at no cost, with no side effects, and with great benefit to the whole body.

DIET—IT'S NOT JUST ABOUT SUGAR

Because diabetes is identified with high blood sugar, most people intuitively think eating sugar causes high blood sugar. They don't know that blood sugar (glucose) is the major source of fuel for our brain and muscles, so just cutting out sugar or all fruit is not going to prevent Type 2 diabetes. A high-fat diet is at the root of the problem in at least two ways. First, it contributes to obesity or being overweight, because high-fat diets tend to be higher in calories; second, fat in the blood makes it more difficult for glucose to get into the muscle to be utilized for energy. Insulin is the hormone that escorts glucose into the muscle. It is now thought that fat blocks the hormone receptors, thus keeping the glucose building up in the blood instead of getting into our muscles.

When the glucose level builds up in our blood, it causes damage to almost every part of the body. Eating the SAD diet causes the blood to get so thick that it can't get into the capillaries. This cuts off circulation to all those parts of the body that rely on these tiny blood vessels to get their blood supply, which provides oxygen, nutrients, and removal of waste products. This damage to diabetics is the leading cause of blindness, neuropathy, kidney disease, and amputations. When the tiny capillaries of the eyes get blocked, vision is damaged—this is how 24,000 Americans go blind every year. When the circulation to the arms and legs is cut off, there is damage to the nerves, which leads to more than 82,000 amputations per year. The same type of damage occurs to the kidneys, which means the kidneys can't do their job of filtering blood. This has led to more than 100,000 dialysis patients or kidney transplants per year in the US alone.[2]

The toll of diabetes is enormous in both economic and human terms. A study published in *Diabetes Care* in March 2003 attributed official estimated costs of diabetes in 2002 at $132 billion, with direct medical costs totaling $92 billion.[3] It was another $40 billion for indirect costs such as absenteeism, restricted activity and disability. Medical costs for diabetics run 2.4 times higher than for non-diabetics. These direct costs have *doubled* between 1997 and 2002. If current trends continue, by the year 2047 the cost will skyrocket to *$32 trillion*, almost triple our present gross domestic product! That's just the dollar costs. The human costs are also horrendous, because as a diabetic becomes physically limited, family and friends have to take up the slack. That's why it's so important to find alternative ways to reverse Type 2 diabetes.

GETTING OFF INSULIN COMPLETELY

I discovered how powerful diet and exercise were in diabetes prevention by accident. I was working with a family whose father had just had a heart attack. The father was willing and ready to change his diet after finding out that a vegan diet could reverse heart disease. I explained to the mother, the cook in the family, the new way of shopping and food preparation they would need. She said that there was no way she was going to prepare two different sets of meals and that the rest of the family was just going to have to eat vegan as well. When I saw the mother a week later, she could hardly contain her enthusiasm. She told me that she was diabetic and on 100 units of insulin a day. After changing her diet for her husband, she started having to lower her insulin. This continued each day and, coupled with going for walks with her husband, by the end of the week she was off insulin completely! (It's too bad that this story did not make the headlines of this morning's newspaper instead of that ad looking for more people to put on drugs.) In addition to having her diabetes reversed, the mother also significantly lowered her own risk of heart disease, hypertension, blindness, neuropathy, loss of her kidneys, amputation, and more. The same diet and exercise program that reverses Type 2 diabetes and heart disease can also affect so many other disease conditions.

Another major risk with diabetes is that, of all the drug dosage errors made in hospitals in this country, the greatest number of errors is made with insulin.[4] This is understandable, because trying to figure out the right amount to administer can be very tricky. The dosage needed is constantly changing, depending on what one eats and the level of exercise. Too much or too little can be life threatening.

EXERCISE CAN HELP IN TWO WAYS

An effective exercise program can help by preventing obesity. By exercising on a daily basis, you greatly diminish your chances of becoming overweight. Furthermore, exercise makes muscles receptive to glucose (blood sugar). There is a condition called "insulin resistance." This occurs when muscles don't get enough exercise and the insulin levels become inadequate to push the glucose into the muscles. Moreover, if the muscles are not contracting, they don't "need" glucose, so it builds up in the blood, doing damage to arterial walls and nerves. Insulin resistance is difficult to measure directly, and it can occur whether or not the level of glucose in the blood is normal. Exercise serves to increase the sensitivity of the muscle cell receptors and lets the insulin open the doors to muscle cells, so to speak, allowing the glucose in. However, you've got to be *using* those muscles for this to work. This is why an effective exercise program is so important.

STOPPING DIABETES IN YOUR GRANDCHILDREN

According to the Centers for Disease Control and Prevention, one in three US children born in 2000 will develop diabetes if they follow current lifestyle habits. In order to avoid this, they have to change their eating and sedentary habits. You can educate them on more healthy habits. We have to get kids off fast food, animal products, and sodas, and get them away from the TV or computer and out running and playing active games.

You may have noted that this chapter addressed only Type 2 diabetes. That's because more than ninety percent of diabetics are in the Type 2 category, and because we know that lifestyle plays the most important role in getting and/or reversing this disease. Type 1 diabetes is a completely different story and does not really fit into senior fitness, because this type occurs when children are young. You need to know, however, that cow's milk appears to be the culprit in causing this autoimmune disease. It is for this reason that children should avoid cow's milk completely.

BOTTOM LINE—WHAT WE KNOW FOR SURE

Diabetes rates are increasing at alarming rates, and we know that Type 2 diabetes is a lifestyle-related disease. Changing to a low-fat vegan diet and getting daily, vigorous exercise is the best way to prevent and even reverse most cases of diabetes.

CHAPTER 10

OSTEOPOROSIS

THE ADMONITIONS SURROUND us. You can't miss all the advertising. "Get more calcium to prevent osteoporosis!" Turn on the TV and you'll see how the antacids will "cure your heartburn and provide calcium, something your body needs anyway." Full-page ads in medical journals show illustrations of a woman through all stages of life, growing tall and then shrinking into an osteoporotic-withered shell. These are followed by pleas to physicians: "Get your patients to drink milk so this won't happen to them."

Osteoporosis is diagnosed when "the bone fractures in a situation that would not normally cause damage to the skeleton" or, more generally, when bone mass decreases for any reason. Age is the factor most commonly associated with bone loss, and the rate of bone loss is highest in post-menopausal women.[1] In spite of what you may have heard, you can build or increase your bone mass after the age of forty-five. I know, because I did it.

HOW MUCH CALCIUM IS ENOUGH?

The most important part of understanding how to build your bone mass is to shatter the myth that osteoporosis is strictly a calcium-deficiency disease. Eskimos, for example, get up to 2,500 mg of calcium per day (way above the RDA or Recommended Daily Allowance) and have the highest rates of osteoporosis in the world.[2] *The British Medical Journal* published a two-part article in 1989 reviewing all the literature on calcium and calcium supplementation and concluded that calcium supplementation was "not justified" at all.[3] Some, however, still cling to the idea that calcium deficiency is a major problem and can cite studies to back their positions as well. I hope to convince you otherwise.

If you wonder how much calcium you need daily, you'll find that recommendations keep changing and it will depend on where you look. The RDA for the US is higher than other countries, reflecting the higher rates of osteoporosis. It had been set at 800 mg a day, but as the incidence of osteoporosis has increased, the US RDA has risen.[4] Depending on which doctor you ask, you'll see recommendations of 1,000 mg, 1,200 mg, 1,500 mg, or even 2,000 mg, especially if you're a post-menopausal female.[5] Even as our RDA has increased, however, we have not seen a decrease in the rates of osteoporosis. What follows is the evidence that the recommendation simply to increase your intake of calcium to prevent osteoporosis is a misguided effort.

Because most people are ethnocentric (meaning they can't see beyond their country's borders), few Americans are aware that osteoporosis is not a big problem in other countries. If you look at the worldwide incidence of osteoporosis, you find that the higher the dairy consumption, the higher the hip fracture rate. Conversely, the countries that don't consume dairy have very low rates of osteoporosis; many have calcium intakes as low as

300–400 mg/day.[6] As with other correlational studies, this does not *prove* a causal relationship. However, it definitely points us in the direction of diet when considered with all the other evidence we now have. So why isn't osteoporosis prevalent in those countries where so little calcium is consumed? Genes are often listed as an answer. However, while there *could* be skeletal and metabolic differences between groups of people, migration studies indicate otherwise.[7] The real paradox is that the higher the calcium intake, in many cases (for instance, the Eskimos' 2,500 mg per day), the higher the bone loss.[8] It turns out that the amount of calcium we need depends on what else we are putting into our bodies.

A SYMPHONY OF MINERALS

Determining the cause of osteoporosis is complicated by the presence of many variables. Those of us who don't use dairy products get our calcium from plant foods. According to the USDA tables, it's highest in green leafy vegetables.[9] Indeed, according to an article published by Heaney and Weaver in the *American Journal of Clinical Nutrition* in 1990, "Greens such as kale [are] . . . at least as good as milk in terms of calcium absorbability."[10] Plus—and this is a big plus—the gut absorbs more calcium when it needs more. Pumping the gut full of calcium pills increases absorption very little and interferes with the absorption of other minerals by blocking the absorption sites.

If you listened to all the advertisements, you'd think that bone was pure calcium. Actually, bone is made of other minerals as well: manganese, fluorine, potassium, zinc, phosphorus, boron, copper, strontium, and more.[11] It's rather like a symphony where each musician has a different part to play and all the instruments have to be properly balanced. You will find this balance of minerals in leafy green vegetables.

ENTER A MAJOR CULPRIT

Most of us know that protein is made of amino acids. The typical omnivore's diet provides excessive protein that then has to be neutralized or buffered. What is overlooked is that acid is, not surprisingly, acidic, and that the sulfur amino acids (SAAs) have an especially acidic pH. Animal protein is much higher in SAAs than plant protein, and it's the SAAs that leach calcium from the bones. If you eat a diet high in animal protein, your blood needs a buffer to handle all the sulfur amino acids, and this buffer comes from your bones.[12] Because plant protein is low in SAAs, consumption of excess plant protein is not considered as problematic.[13] However, in an email he wrote to me, Dr. John McDougall explained, "It is the bicarbonate released from the bone and other alkaline materials that do the neutralizing. Also, plant proteins can be a problem if they are artificial and concentrated like seitan and Isolated Soy Protein. Plus, I would limit the amount of legumes (beans) and grains in the diet of someone with osteoporosis."[14]

Meat Is High in Acid

Compare the acid load* of various foods
(renal acid load per 100 calories)

Beef 6.3
Chicken 7.0
Fish (cod) 9.3
Cheddar cheese 10.0

Peas 1.0
Wheat flour 1.0
Potatoes -5.0
Apples -5.0
Banana -6.0

Tomatoes -18.0
Spinach -56.0

*a measure of acidity or alkalinity where positive num-
bers indicate acid-producing foods and negative numbers indicate alkaline-producing foods

Figure 1. Meat and other animal products have much higher sulfur amino acid amounts than vegetable foods, including beans and grains. You can calculate this yourself using J Pennington. *Bowes & Church's Food Values of Portions Commonly Used,* 17th ed. (Philadelphia, New York: Lippincott, 1998). Be sure to make calculations based on calories consumed (not weight of food).

We also see a positive correlation of osteoporosis with lifestyle factors such as smoking;[15] drinking coffee,[16] alcohol, and sodas; long-term use of steroids;[17] sodium from prepared or animal foods; and a sedentary lifestyle.[18]

THE SECOND CULPRIT

Possibly the major cause of osteoporosis is lack of effective exercise. In order to understand this, you should consider how we build muscle. No matter how much protein powder you take, no muscle will pop up to build you bulging biceps unless you start an effective weight-lifting program. In fact, protein powders may contribute to bone *loss* (as well as kidney damage), since most protein powders contain egg whites, casein, and whey—all animal proteins high in sulfur amino acids.

To build muscle, you need to put stress on it. If you gradually put more stress on a muscle than it is accustomed to handling, it responds by adding more muscle. As more weight is added, the muscle gets bigger. The same is true of bone. Bone is much like muscle in that it only gets as strong (dense) as the demands placed on it. No matter how much calcium you take, no bone will be built unless you apply effective stress to the bone, assuming normal hormone levels. Later, we'll be discussing the role of the hormone progesterone in building bone in postmenopausal women, who don't have normal hormone levels, but for most people, effective exercise is the critical factor in building bones. Good evidence of this is in the bone density of tennis players. The dominant arm has about thirty-five percent greater bone density, and, obviously, both arms get the same amount of calcium.[19]

Demands in the form of stress range in a continuum from zero gravity in space to bed-rest, sitting, standing, walking, running, and jumping (the highest-impact stress). Therefore, runners have greater bone density than walkers, and walkers have greater bone density than people convalescing in bed, and people in bed have greater bone density than astronauts—since even gravity can make a significant difference in bone density. Astronauts in space lose two percent of their bone mass per month. Shannon Lucid, the then fifty-three-year-old woman who returned from 188 days in space, logged 2.7 hours a day exercising and was able to walk off her spacecraft instead of being carried, as the others had to be.

BEYOND WALKING

Many people are told to get their exercise through walking. Evidence suggests, however, that walking does not stress the bones enough to stimulate bone growth or even prevent bone loss.[20] The low impact generated by walking is frequently inadequate to reach the threshold of stimulation to bones. High impact, on the other hand, builds bone by sending tiny electric shocks (the piezo-electric effect) to the bone cells, which stimulates the osteoblasts to lay down new bone. Kenneth Cooper, MD, calls this "striking," which he believes is necessary to build bones. This is why running is so effective and why I believe that "impact," which so many believe is a problem in bone wellness, is really what keeps bones strong and even makes them stronger. Striking—for example in running—works because every time the foot strikes with the impact of one's compounded weight, it involves the repeated transfer of energy through the bones and joints and stimulates more bone challenge and growth. As mentioned in the chapter on exercise, this same mechanism helps maintain joint cartilage.

Women aged forty to eighty who claim to have done everything that was recommended by their doctors are being diagnosed with osteoporosis. I hear from many women who have taken "lots" of calcium (usually in the form of low-fat dairy products such as skim milk) and walk for twenty minutes three times a week, yet have been told they have osteoporosis. They are feeling angry and betrayed by the "system" and the fact they weren't given good medical advice. Walking can sometimes maintain bone density, but it does not increase it. Only running and jumping have been shown to actually increase bone density—where quality trumps quantity. It's really a concept involving a continuum from zero gravity to the greatest impact generated by landing on one foot after a high jump. The way most people walk does not generate enough force or stress to accomplish the desired result.

BEYOND ESTROGEN

Although it is true that estrogen temporarily slows down the activities of the osteoclasts (the cells that remove old bone), it does not stop bone loss. Once the estrogen is stopped, a "catching up" effect seems to occur and bone loss is accelerated.[21] John Lee, MD, prescribed natural progesterone cream to his patients, and as a result their bone mass increased by as much as forty percent.[22] Progesterone seems to stimulate the osteoblasts (the cells that build new bone). Conversely, progestin (synthetic progesterone), which is very different from natural progesterone, not only does not increase bone density, but also causes a whole host of negative side effects.[23]

Alendronate and non-hormonal bone-building drugs act by slowing down the rate of bone remodeling, or the activity of the osteoclasts. Bones show increased density in the short term, but they are more brittle, so it appears that, over the long term, these drugs will not lower the rate of hip fractures.[24]

INCREASING BONE DENSITY AFTER FIFTY

In my own case, I was diagnosed with breast cancer at the same time my menopause started at the age of forty-seven. Because of a strong history of osteoporosis on both sides of my family, I've been monitored very closely. To give you some perspective on what has happened to me since, you need to know that the average thirty-year-old female has a bone density of 411 mg/cm^2—theoretically, her peak bone mass.[25] Here are my results: At age fifty, my bone density was 447, already way above the statistical average. However, by age sixty, my bone density had increased to 466! I attribute the increase to my change to a vegan diet at age forty-seven and a strenuous exercise program—doing Ironman Triathlons, averaging fifty to sixty races a year, and daily running since age thirty-three. I have this high bone density despite ingesting no dairy products, no calcium supplements, and no estrogen since the onset of menopause. It's worth repeating that I have a strong history of osteoporosis on *both* sides of my family, so it's not my genes.

FALLING DOWN

Falls are inevitable, and most of the time, people get up, dust themselves off, and go on about their business. However, when you get older, the scenario changes. People eating the SAD diet and getting little or no exercise are much more prone to falling. Indeed, one in three people over the age of sixty-five suffer falls each year.[26]

These falls are sometimes the result (rather than the cause) of breaking a bone in the hip, frequently just below the head of the femur. As I have suggested, we lose bone density gradually because we eat a diet high in protein and place inadequate stress on our bones to maintain their strength. Over a period of years, this reaches the point where the bone can't support the weight of the body. A lack of exposure to sunshine also plays a role, in that Vitamin D may be deficient; this can be an important factor for those living in the higher latitudes or who are housebound. Such people need to ensure some regular source of Vitamin D.

The consequences from a fall can be deadly. One in two women and one in three men will suffer a bone-density-related fracture in their lifetime. One in four will die within six months, and two in four will never get out of bed, requiring long-term nursing care. What we are not told, however, is that of the deaths studied, most were over eighty-five and were close to dying anyway, given their other ailments. Of those who were active and walking before the fracture, fewer than fourteen percent of the deaths following the fracture were attributed to the hip or pelvic fracture.[27]

In general, falling is frequently the marker for frail health and is many times aggravated by the fact that older people may be on drugs such as corticosteroids (which weaken bones), antipsychotics, and powerful, long-acting tranquilizers. In any case, the treatment is obvious. It's not drugs and surgery, but a low-fat vegan diet and gradually increasing, effective exercise that will diminish the chances of osteoporosis. I also recommend the balancing exercises described in a later chapter to maintain and improve your equilibrium.

THE MARKETING OF OSTEOPOROSIS

In the early 1980s, most women had never heard of osteoporosis, and most doctors saw few patients with the disease. By 1982, however, a major promotional campaign sponsored by a large pharmaceutical company had as its mission (a very successful one, I might add) to create an awareness of this "disease."[28] This company also happened to be the major producer of Premarin, a drug that delivers estrogen obtained from the urine of pregnant horses. It was thought at the time that menopause caused a rapid loss of bone density and that Premarin was the solution to the problem by slowing bone loss. There was a massive advertising campaign on radio and television, and in magazines and medical journals. Because the campaign was so effective, women went in droves to their doctors to be put on estrogen. The dairy and calcium supplement industries jumped on the bandwagon, seeing the opportunity to link osteoporosis with a milk or calcium deficiency.

After this came the development of the Dual X-ray Absorptiometry (DXA) scan, developed to measure bone density. DXA has become the gold standard for determining osteoporosis risk, even though bone density is not the only factor contributing to fractures. As it turns out, bone density is not a good predictor of fracture risk.[29] In other words, men and women with low bone density are *not* more likely to fracture than those with high bone density.

Another variable comes with the standardization of the DXA tests. Using twenty-year-olds as your reference standard, you will increase the "patient" load immeasurably since most people do not exercise enough to maintain bone density as they age. Once a person is told she has low bone density, she is subjected to a lifetime of bone density tests, radiation, drugs, and fear of doing anything strenuous—just the opposite of what she should be doing. Incidentally, the loss of height is a good measurement of osteoporosis, and in the chapter on motivation I cover a number of tests you can do yourself, one of which is a test for osteoporosis you can easily do at home.

The drug companies have joined forces with the bone-density-measuring companies. In 1995, two of the largest suppliers of DXA scans formed an alliance with Merck. Merck produces Fosamax (alendronate), a drug that according to the trade magazine *Medical Devices & Diagnostic Magazine* netted Merck $1.3 billion dollars in 2000.[30] Vulnerable men and women are easy targets for the persuasive marketing strategies of the drug companies, the medical devices sales, the medical profession, and the calcium and dairy industries.

BOTTOM LINE—WHAT WE KNOW FOR SURE

First, aging doesn't mean automatic bone loss. The evidence suggests we don't have to lose bone mass as we age. With a whole-food, high-leafy-green vegan diet and lots of effective exercise, we can maintain or even increase bone density. Last, we know that we've got pretty smart bodies—just give them the right fuel and remember this about "dem bones": use 'em or lose 'em!

CHAPTER 11

ARTHRITIS—DIET *DOES* MAKE A DIFFERENCE

T HE WORD "ARTHRO" means "joint," while "-itis" means inflammation. There are more than a hundred types of arthritis, the two most common being osteo- and rheumatoid arthritis. The other less common types include lupus, fibromyalgia, scleroderma, polymyalgia, and juvenile arthritis. They are classed as autoimmune diseases, meaning the body's antibodies are turning against it. Those of us who are aware that diet can reverse the inflammation think the body does this because our antibodies are overzealous and confuse our own protein with foreign (animal) protein.[1] When you stop ingesting animal protein, the antibodies settle down and the inflammation disappears. This diet and exercise regimen, I believe, is certainly worth a try for any of the types of arthritis.

Why our antibodies behave this way is a mystery. However, it is thought that autoimmune disease sufferers have an abnormality of the digestive tract called "leaky gut syndrome." This involves damage to the gut lining that allows large protein molecules of incompletely digested food particles to pass through the intestinal wall into the bloodstream.[2] William Harris, MD, has shown that there is a strong correlation between the consumption of animal protein and musculoskeletal diseases, including autoimmune diseases.[3] He also shows an inverse correlation between consumption of plant foods and musculoskeletal diseases, meaning that people who eat a diet of vegetables and fruits lower their risk of these diseases.[4]

Most people, when diagnosed with arthritis, are immediately put on anti-inflammatory drugs. They are told that arthritis is progressive and irreversible and that they will have to take these drugs for the rest of their lives. Despite what most people have heard, you *can* frequently stop and even sometimes even reverse the damage done by arthritis using the same two components that we have shown affect most other afflictions: diet and exercise.

The most common type of arthritis, osteoarthritis, is known as "degenerative" arthritis or the "wear and tear" type of arthritis. Intuitively, it may seem that as we age our joints would wear out. However, while that might be true if you were to reach two hundred years of age, it's certainly not true for people reaching their fifties, sixties, seventies, and eighties, when joint replacement has become so common.

On the face of it, it may seem that in osteoarthritis the cartilage has "worn out," or joints have become red, painful, and swollen and have outlived their usefulness. In most cases, however, arthritis is caused by foreign (usually animal) proteins getting caught in the joint capsule. The body's usual response to a foreign protein is to create inflammation (the typical redness, pain, and swelling symptoms).[5] The typical medical approach in the West after the diagnosis of osteoarthritis is to put the patient on an anti-inflammatory drug, which treats the symptom but not the underlying problem. When I was diagnosed with osteoarthritis a few years before my breast cancer diagnosis, the rheumatologist told me that my osteoarthritis was progressive and irreversible but that I was "lucky" because a new anti-inflammatory drug had just come on the market that would really help. He wrote out a prescription for Naprosyn, naproxen or Aleve—all different names for the same drug.

I will be the first to admit that the drug really *did* relieve the symptoms. After taking it for four years, however, I landed in the emergency room with acute gastrointestinal bleeding. This happened to be the year after my breast cancer diagnosis and the change to my vegan diet. I was forced to stop the Naprosyn, of course, and that was when Dr. John McDougall told me that I needn't find another anti-inflammatory because, as he said, "Your arthritis went away when you changed your diet." Sure enough, it had. In my experience, taking an anti-inflammatory drug is not the answer to beating osteoarthritis; avoiding the foreign protein is.

THE ROLE OF DIET

Because the damage done to cartilage can progress to the point where you see bone on bone on the x-ray, it is usually assumed that the damage is irreversible. This is also supported by the fact that cartilage has a limited blood supply and therefore heals very slowly. However, you need to know that that is not necessarily the end of the story.

As you might imagine, a tiny piece of a cow, pig, chicken, or fish getting caught in the joint capsule would cause a major rejection response. After all, just think about what happens when a closely related protein from another *human* gets into our bodies. Massive rejection! People have actually died when medical mistakes such as a human tissue mismatch occurs and the wrong kidney or heart gets transplanted. Even with a good match, people with transplants have to take anti-rejection drugs for the rest of their lives to keep their bodies from rejecting the foreign human tissue. If our bodies are so sensitive to other *human* tissue, why should we not expect them to be as sensitive to tissue from a cow, pig, fish, or bird?

We have already discussed how pieces of flesh pass through the intestinal wall (leaky gut syndrome), into the bloodstream, and into a joint. The good news is that the process is reversible; if you stop eating animal foods, the inflammation dies down and the arthritis may be gone forever.

EXERCISE IS NECESSARY TO KEEP JOINTS HEALTHY

Orthopedists know that exercise is crucial to maintain joint health. In fact, joints need to be put through their entire range of motion at least once every twenty-four hours. Otherwise, adhesions start forming that eventually lead to a so-called "frozen" joint.[6] The formation of restrictive adhesions around the joint after injury is one of the most vexing processes faced by physicians and rehabilitation specialists.

Exercise provides much of that range of motion, but it also provides another important factor in maintaining joint health, and that is muscular strength. The muscles above and below each joint are responsible for maintaining the weight of the body and keep it from damaging the joint. For example, the knee is a joint that is frequently damaged because the muscles of the upper leg don't do their job of supporting the weight of the body. Exercise is important in keeping both the knee and the upper leg strong. Studies show that athletes such as marathon runners do not get arthritis any more frequently than non-runners, something that should put to rest the myth that running is hard on the joints.[7] Runners actually have thicker knee cartilage than sedentary people.

RHEUMATOID ARTHRITIS

What applies to osteoarthritis applies to rheumatoid arthritis (RA) as well. The main difference between RA and osteoarthritis is that the condition of RA involves the lining around the joint becoming inflamed. This inflammation increases the level of fluid in the joint and leads to thickening of the lining. Moving or touching the joint causes pain and eventually leads to deformation and destruction of the joint.

For years, it was thought that exercise would damage the joints of people with RA. However, research conducted by Leiden University Medical Center in the Netherlands showed that long-term, high-intensity exercise benefited people with early-stage RA, both physically and mentally.[8] Researchers took three hundred people with RA and assigned them either to an intensive exercise program or to regular physical therapy. The study participants all met twice a week, but the high-exercise group performed twenty minutes of strength training with weights, twenty minutes of stationary cycling with a heart rate maximum of between seventy and ninety percent, and twenty minutes of a sport of their choice (usually basketball, volleyball, or soccer), while the others underwent regular physical therapy. After two years, the group that had exercised heavily had significantly greater improvement in the functional ability of, and no increase in damage to, their joints. They also experienced less anxiety and depression.

In another study with RA patients, John McDougall, MD, John Westerdahl, Ph.D, RD, and others put RA patients on a low-fat vegan diet and found that the symptoms of pain lessened significantly, while blood tests verified that the inflammation had decreased.[9]

AVOIDING JOINT REPLACEMENT

As technology improves, more and more people resort to joint replacement. However, no artificial knee, hip, or other joint will function as well as the original equipment, as long you take good care of it. Artificial joints will not last as long as your need for them. This is why younger people with deteriorating joints are sometimes made to wait until their joint gets so bad that they just cannot function. If only they were told to change their diet and start a daily, vigorous exercise program, they could reverse that decline in functional ability and be less likely to need a joint replacement.

PREVENTING AND REDUCING
LOWER BACK PAIN

Most back pain that is diagnosed as arthritis is also due to poor lifestyle practices involving both diet and exercise. In the September 1995 issue of the *Lancet*, Leena Kauppila wrote that back disease is actually caused by artery disease, similar to the process that occurs in a heart attack or stroke.[10] Each vertebra and disc receives blood from arteries that arise in the aorta. When people eat the SAD diet, we know that atherosclerosis of the arteries increases; this illness is found in people with degenerative disc disease. In fact, studies have shown that people with back pain on average have two blocked arteries in their lower back.[11] Atherosclerosis is reversible, and many people, including myself, have found relief from chronic back pain by changing to a low-fat vegan diet. Exercises such as regular running strengthen the lower back muscles that help support the vertebrae and discs.

THE DANGERS OF ANTI-INFLAMMATORIES

Most research shows that anti-inflammatory drugs, while masking the pain, actually make arthritis worse. This is another case of disabling the alarm system instead of putting out the fire. The pain and stiffness of a joint disappear, but people continue eating the foods and following the lifestyle that is causing their arthritic joints to inflame and deteriorate. Anti-inflammatories and the new COX-2 inhibitors also have many side effects.[12] I know several people who have landed in the hospital from the gastrointestinal bleeding that these drugs cause. As I have stated many times already, it is far better to eliminate the cause of disease in the first place.

BOTTOM LINE—WHAT WE KNOW FOR SURE

Eating a low-fat vegan diet and getting daily, vigorous exercise can reverse most cases of arthritis. Exercise is necessary to protect and increase circulation to the joints and will build stronger muscles to help support the joints.

CHAPTER 12

HYPERTENSION AND DVTS

H IGH BLOOD PRESSURE, or hypertension as it's known medically, is a major problem in this country—and it just got bigger. Millions of people who thought they had safe blood pressure levels are now being told that what was considered "borderline" is now considered too high. The new federal guidelines say blood pressure readings of 120/80 to 139/90 are too high and are considered "pre-hypertension." The National Heart, Lung and Blood Institute in 2003 announced these new guidelines because of the recognition that blood pressure in these ranges increases the risk of stroke, heart failure and kidney disease.[1] Forty-five million Americans are affected, providing a huge potential market for the drug companies. What people don't know is that, for most people, simple changes in the diet and the addition of an exercise program will lower their blood pressure.

DIET—IT'S NOT JUST ABOUT SALT

Most people, when told they have hypertension or high blood pressure, are also told they need to cut down on their salt intake. What they are *not* told is that most people's high blood pressure is not just about the salt. But they go home, follow instructions to stop using the salt shaker, and go back to their doctor's office a couple of weeks later. When their blood pressure is still high, they are told that they have to go on medication. What they should be told is that most people are not salt-sensitive, and if they had been put on a low-fat vegan diet and started an effective exercise program, their blood pressure would probably drop into the normal range very quickly.[2]

EXERCISE

According to studies, one bout of exercise lowers blood pressure for twenty-four hours.[3] That's the good news. The "bad news" is that you have to do this every day! This is "bad news" to most people; if you're fit and healthy, it's "good news"! This method of controlling blood pressure has so many other advantages that I hope you've integrated exercise into your daily schedule like brushing your teeth and combing your hair. You'd never think about skipping tooth and hair care; likewise, you should never think about skipping your health care.

DEEP VEIN THROMBOSIS

Deep Vein Thrombosis (DVT) came to public attention when it was noticed that, on occasion, people who had been sitting in an airplane for long flights got off the plane, collapsed and died. Blood clots had formed in their legs, and when they got up the clots traveled to their lungs, a potentially fatal condition called pulmonary embolism. This can be fatal. DVT came to be known as the "economy class syndrome."[4]

DVT and pulmonary embolism have also reportedly occurred in persons taking plane trips as short as three to four hours. It was speculated that the low cabin humidity and/or alcohol intake contributed to this condition. The clots can also do their damage several days after a flight, so people are now encouraged to get up more frequently to increase the circulation of blood in their legs, drink nonalcoholic drinks at regular intervals, and avoid smoking.

The above factors undoubtedly are significant in the onset of DVT. One contributor to this condition, however, is very likely the stickiness of blood cells consequent to eating a high-fat meal.[5] Animal fats cause clumping of the blood cells, whereas plant fats do not.[6] This condition can also occur any time one sits or lies down for an extended period of time—for example, at one's desk, on a long drive in a car, or during surgery. Vegans tend to have thin blood and meat-eaters thick, sludgy blood. Avoiding DVT is another good reason to eat a low-fat vegan diet.

HOW TO AVOID TAKING DRUGS

So-called "blood thinners," such as coumadin (warfarin) and heparin, are among the most frequently prescribed drugs in this country. These drugs are prescribed because, as stated earlier, diets high in fat and full of animal products tend to thicken the blood. So, instead of getting to the cause of the problem, physicians will generally just write a prescription. Blood thinners are not without serious risks, however, since they can lead to hemorrhages and bleeding that can be fatal. Wouldn't it be smarter to just get at the cause of the thick, sludgy blood?

I know one very smart senior who did just that. As I write

this, sixty-year-old Bob Leitch is celebrating a birthday today—actually, a vegan rebirth day. In the winter of 1996 and then again in the winter of 1997, Bob suffered bouts of DVT and was hospitalized both times; both times he was put on coumadin to thin his blood. After the second bout, which was more serious than the first, his doctor told him he could never come off the coumadin again—that this time, he would have to stay on it for life. This really upset Bob, and he started looking for a better way to deal with his DVT. When I, Dr. John McDougall, and Dr. William Harris confirmed that switching to a low-fat vegan diet would thin his blood, he tried it, staying under a physician's care. Bob's physician said that he doubted it would work, and asked him to at least take a daily aspirin.

After six months of excellent blood readings, Bob's doctor told him that his blood work was so good that he didn't even have to take aspirin any more. In addition to the diet thinning his blood and allowing him to get off coumadin, Bob discovered an amazing number of other benefits. The morning after changing his diet, he found to his delight that his chronic constipation had disappeared. Because he was an asthmatic and a runner and always had to take his "puffer" with him, Bob soon discovered that his asthma had disappeared. Then the "lesion" on his prostate that was concerning both Bob and his urologist started vanishing. The next thing that went was about sixty pounds of fat, which Bob lost without even trying. The weight loss was a very pleasant surprise, as was the end of Bob's headaches that were so frequent they had caused him to become addicted to codeine. If you were to ask Bob if he'd ever go back to his old meat-eating ways, he'd look at you as if you were crazy. Plus, he's too busy celebrating his sixth vegan birthday. (One word of caution. If you are on blood thinners, be sure to do as Bob did and not drop the medications without having a physician monitor your blood.)

BOTTOM LINE—WHAT WE KNOW FOR SURE

To avoid high blood pressure, DVTs, and the need for blood thinners, eat a low-fat vegan diet and get daily, vigorous exercise.

CHAPTER 13

Obesity—This Epidemic *Can* Be Controlled

As public health experts and politicians finally recognize how serious it is that such a large number of people in the United States are obese and overweight, everyone is finding someone or something to blame. Some accuse the fast food industry and oversized food portions, while others blame the amount of fat or carbohydrates in the food. Some say that our sedentary lifestyle is at fault, while others suggest that our genes are the problem. Meanwhile, weight loss gimmicks in the form of pills and diets galore promise quick and easy weight loss. Turn on the television, and you'll see lots of infomercials for weight loss equipment costing from hundreds to thousands of dollars.

Yet very few public officials or medical organizations have advocated a diet without animal foods and rich in fruits and vegetables. The reasons, you will not be surprised to hear, are that there is no money to be made in such a dietary change and that eating animals is deeply entrenched in our culture.

I indicated earlier in the book that if you eat the foods that most Americans eat, you'll get the diseases that most Americans get. This is certainly true with regard to obesity. If you eat the foods most Americans eat, you'll have the same high risk of obesity that most Americans face—and currently, *two thirds* of all Americans are overweight or obese. Most Americans eat lots of animal products, which are very high in fat, and very little in the way of fresh fruits and vegetables, which are very low in caloric density. The simple truth is that it is almost impossible to be overweight on a diet rich in fruits and vegetables.

Just as obesity is very simply the result of taking in more calories than you burn, weight loss is also very simply the burning of more calories than you take in. Not many people will pay you a lot of money for that advice, however, whereas they seem quite willing to pay a lot of money for diet books, pills, drinks, and any gimmick that promises quick and easy weight loss.

This whole chapter could be summed up by the following: "Eat as much as you want of a low-fat vegan diet and you will take in fewer calories and not be hungry; start daily running or similar activity and you will start burning calories at a high rate and lose weight." This is also a program that you can stay on for life!

HOW TO TELL IF YOU'RE OBESE

A straightforward measure of the appropriate weight-to-height ratio is the Body Mass Index (BMI). BMI is calculated as your weight in kilograms divided by the square of your height in meters. For those of us who do not think in meters and kilograms, there's an easy way to figure BMI. Get a calculator and follow along.

- First, figure your height in inches, then multiply that number by itself. If you're 5′ 8″, for instance, you're 68 inches tall: 68 x

68 equals 4,624. Next, divide your weight by that number. So if you weigh 125 pounds, that means: 125 divided by 4,624 equals .0270328.

- Now, multiply that last number by 703. In the case of our example, that equals 19.00. That number is your BMI. If that really *is* your BMI, then you and I are both at the low range of the "normal" zone, as those are my figures, too.

A BMI of 18.5 to 24.9 is normal. Overweight is 25.0 to 29.9. A BMI of 30.0 or above is considered obese.

These BMI ranges are used to determine relative risk for certain diseases such as heart disease, cancer, stroke, and Type 2 diabetes.[1] According to recent research from Utah State University, women who have BMIs in the obese range or the upper end of the overweight range may be at considerably higher risk of developing Alzheimer's disease as they age.[2] (See Chapter 15.)

Obesity is at epidemic proportions in this country today and continues to worsen every year. Obese people have an increased risk of high blood pressure, heart disease, diabetes, gallstones, cancer of several different types, arthritis, and even sleep apnea (in which a person stops breathing temporarily because of all the fat around his throat and chest), which can lead to a heart attack or stroke. According to the Centers for Disease Control and Prevention, obese people are at fifty to one hundred percent greater risk of dying prematurely.[3] Psychologically, of course, obesity is devastating to one's self-esteem and can lead to isolation and severe depression. Unfortunately, many obese people have tried countless diets and still don't lose weight. Studies have shown that even with significant weight loss, they are likely to gain all the weight back and then some.

Most people who are fighting obesity are told that obesity is the *cause* of heart disease, cancer, stroke, etc. and that this is the reason they should lose weight. There is a big gap in critical thinking here, in that obesity itself is not actually the major problem. What *is* the problem is that an animal-based, high-fat diet causes both the obesity and these diseases. Simply losing weight will not prevent you from getting heart disease and cancer, although it may certainly help. Too many people in this country with low or ideal body weights still get heart attacks and cancer. They get the heart attacks and cancer because animal foods are directly related to the causes of heart disease, cancer, and, of course, the other diseases discussed in this book. By changing to a low-fat vegan diet, your weight goes down along with your risk of disease.

Approximately six thousand people die every day from complications from obesity, and there is much at stake in finding a quick answer to reversing this epidemic.[4] Research scientists and drug companies are searching frantically for a medical treatment for obesity. There are hundreds of drugs and hormones being investigated to see if they are the "magic bullet" that will reverse obesity. There are billions of dollars to be made because of all the people who are seeking that "magic bullet"—weight loss in a pill. Gastric bypass surgery has become a very common operation, with people even trying to gain weight to meet the requirements set by the surgeon for this very drastic treatment for obesity.

Surgery is now considered an option for those with a body mass index (BMI) of over forty—which is about eighty pounds overweight for women or 100 pounds for men—and when all other non-surgical means have been tried and have failed. However, there can be a number of very serious side effects to the surgery. These include malabsorption (food passing too quickly for the nutrients to be absorbed), vomiting (if food is not chewed adequately), dumping (again, food passing too quickly, in this case leading to weakness, nausea, sweating, fainting, or diarrhea), gallstones, and severe lifestyle changes, including special foods, medication, and close medical supervision.

There have been best-selling weight-loss books on the market for forty to fifty years now. Yet, while low-calorie diets will produce weight loss, when the person goes off the diet, the fat comes back, plus about twenty percent more. Look at the past and present bestseller lists and you will see almost every variation of diet. There are high-protein/low-carb diets, and the opposite, low-protein/high-carb diets. There are low-fat and high-fat diets, and, occasionally, a moderate approach to protein, carbs, and fat.

All these diets, with their various gimmicks, have one thing in common: They are designed to limit the number of calories you consume. What we know is that going on a diet that just limits calories is not a successful strategy for long-term weight loss. What *is* successful is to allow people to eat as much as they want of whole vegetables and fruits. This is also the healthiest diet. All the other diets are inherently unhealthy—except for the low-protein/high-carb diet, if it eliminates animal foods, processed and refined foods, and oils, and does not restrict vegetables and fruit.

CHOOSING THE RIGHT FOODS
AND EXERCISE

Because of the epidemic of obesity, there has been much discussion about diets and weight loss and how to succeed in losing weight. Cutting calories may seem to be an obvious solution. However, appetites are powerful survival drives and are difficult to deny for very long. Some doctors push diets high in protein and low in carbohydrates in the misguided belief that this will keep insulin levels down and, theoretically, keep calories from turning to fat. Studies show that this is not so. Meat and other high-protein, high-fat foods raise insulin levels just as much and, in some cases, more than carbohydrates.[5] For example, a serving of beef raises insulin levels twenty-seven percent higher than a serving of pasta. The brain, body, and muscles need carbohydrates to run on and will break down muscle if they do not have enough carbohydrates. In addition, as we noted above, while those who go on high-protein diets may lose weight in the beginning, they usually regain all the weight they lost and more.

Other diets promote low-fat eating, because fat has more than twice the number of calories as carbohydrates and protein. One can go astray on these diets, however, by consuming so-called "low-fat" foods, which are often filled with sugar to make them more palatable. This means these foods often have as many *or more* calories than the low-fat foods.

OBESITY IS FROM EATING THE WRONG FOODS

In order to deal with the weight issue sensibly, we need to take the word "diet" out of our vocabulary. Instead, we need to think about eating healthfully. Obesity, after all, is a *symptom* of something wrong with a person's eating habits. It is a function of our mindset that we think of obesity as something to *cure*: In this area, as in so many others, Western medicine treats the symptoms instead of getting to the *cause* of the disorder.

In changing the priority from *losing weight* to *regaining health*, we can start by examining the nutritional charts and looking up the healthiest foods, the ones that rank the highest in nutrient per calorie ratio. These are the leafy greens. Therefore, for the optimum diet, you'll want the number one food you eat to be leafy greens. Since you can't, or wouldn't want to, exist on greens alone, you go to the next highest optimum health foods, which are all the other vegetables. These, therefore, should be your second highest-frequency foods. Again, you probably won't want to exist on just greens and veggies, so you should look for the third highest optimum health foods. These are fruit.

Therefore, your healthiest foods are, in order of nutrient-per-calorie ratio and priority of health-giving benefits, 1) greens, 2) all other veggies, and 3) fruit. This gives you an amazing variety of foods from which to choose. For example, in the standard food tables, there are more than ninety different vegetables and sixty different fruits. When you consider all the different varieties of edible vegetables and fruits, you could try a different dish every day of the year without repeating a single one. It's almost guaranteed that you'll fill up your stomach at every meal and be at your optimum weight for the rest of your long and healthy life. Thus, the secret is to think about eating the healthiest foods and forget about dieting.

Another major advantage to eating the healthiest foods is that you don't ever have to count calories, fat grams, grams of carbohydrate, or worry about getting enough protein or too much cholesterol. This is because, given a variety of whole plant foods as your diet, your appetite is the best guide to how many calories your body needs. You'll also automatically be getting just the right amount of fat, protein, and carbohydrates, with zero grams of cholesterol and lots of fiber to fill you up.

There is one more bit of good news. The healthiest foods are often the cheapest foods, so you save money as well. As of this writing, carrots cost me forty-four cents a pound, cabbage thirty-nine cents, watermelon forty-nine cents (down to ten cents a pound in July), and bananas, as low as nineteen cents a pound in Chinatown. That is inexpensive, healthy eating.

TRYING—AND FAILING—TO LOSE WEIGHT LOWERS MORTALITY

Research suggests that simply *attempting* to lose weight, even if that attempt is unsuccessful, lowers mortality rates substantially. Over 6,000 subjects, all at least thirty-five years of age, were asked to fill out a survey in 1989 regarding their intentions to lose weight.[6] It was found that people who lost weight intentionally had a twenty-four percent drop in mortality, compared with subjects not trying to lose weight and reporting no weight change. For those who lost between two and twenty pounds, the mortality rate dropped even more, by thirty percent. Mortality rates were far lower in people who reported trying to lose weight than in those not trying to lose weight, independent of their actual weight loss. For the unsuccessful weight loss subjects, mortality rates fell an impressive nineteen percent. The best explanation for these findings is that people who are trying to lose weight make healthier food choices and adopt other healthy behaviors, such as exercising, that lower mortality. The lesson is, if you are overweight, keep on trying to get down to a healthy weight, even if you don't succeed.

The story from the survey was very different, however, for people who lost weight unintentionally. Their mortality rate was thirty-one percent higher. Since unintentional weight loss is frequently associated with cancer, heart disease, depression and alcoholism, it clearly needs to be differentiated from intentional weight loss. We know that changing to a low-fat vegan diet can reverse cancer and heart disease, and exercise helps with all these conditions. In some cases, people adopting a low-fat vegan diet lose weight so quickly that they get very concerned. The solution is to eat more. Many people can't believe how much they get to eat when it's a healthful diet of fruits and vegetables. Weight usually stabilizes at a proper level.

EXERCISE IS ALL ABOUT MOVING

In the chapter on exercise, we talked about the importance of exercise in maintaining a strong body. This is even truer as we age, since most people tend to do less as they get older and put on weight. To reverse this effect, we need to make a special effort to increase the amount of exercise we do. I have already addressed the different types of exercise—aerobic, walking, running, etc.—you can do. It doesn't matter which one you pick. All you need to do is to pick an exercise plan and stick with it.

BOTTOM LINE—WHAT WE KNOW FOR SURE

To maintain a healthy weight for the rest of your life, eat a low-fat, whole-food vegan diet and get daily, vigorous exercise. You don't have to worry about counting anything—not calories, not carbs, not fat grams, not anything! You can eat your fill of raw fruits and veggies, never go hungry, save lots of time, and maintain an ideal weight.

CHAPTER 14

Sexy Seniors

THE ROLE OF HORMONES,
MALE AND FEMALE

A WHOLE BOOK could be written about the role of hormones in both behavior and health. However, what you need to know is that most health problems are *not* hormonal in nature. People love to blame their shortcomings on hormones, as if just taking a pill or a shot would "fix" them up. This is especially true among both men and women when they reach their fifties. Women hit menopause and men hit viropause, and entire industries thrive because of the beliefs and false hopes associated with hormonal replacement.

Women are told that hot flashes, insomnia, weight gain, irritability, fluid retention, vaginal dryness, loss of libido, wrinkles, and so on are caused by a drop in their estrogen levels. In actuality, most women's estrogen levels remain quite adequate, and adding more estrogen leads to increased rates of cervical and breast cancer, strokes, and blood clots instead of the promised benefits, lower rates of heart disease and osteoporosis.[1] The results of a large study, the Women's Health Initiative,[2] showed this on such a scale that it was determined to be unethical to continue the study, and it was terminated to get the women off the estrogen/progestin drugs they were on. It was too dangerous to continue to expose them to that high a risk of cancer, strokes, and blood clots.

Unfortunately, after being taken off the hormones, the women were not told that the best solution to their menopausal symptoms was a low-fat vegan diet and lots of effective exercise. For the few for whom the vegan and high-intensity exercise regimen is not enough, natural progesterone usually takes care of the remaining symptoms. (Note that progesterone is very different from the *progestins* given to women in the study and most commonly by doctors in general. This is why we normally refer to it as "natural progesterone," to differentiate it from synthetic progestin. More on that later.)

TESTOSTERONE

Testosterone is the primary sex hormone for men and is responsible for their secondary sex characteristics, such as their deeper voice, facial hair, greater muscle development, aggression, and their sex drive, or libido. Women also have testosterone, albeit at much lower levels, just as men have some estrogen as well. It's the balance that's important—having enough but not too much.

Men are told that their testosterone levels drop as they age and that is the reason for their weight gain, irritability, loss of muscle, and (primarily) loss of libido. Loss of libido can manifest, men are told, in erectile dysfunction (ED), the inability to get or maintain an erection.

Testosterone therapy is an unproven yet growing practice

among aging men that, according to a one-year study by the Institute of Medicine, urgently needs closer study to establish its benefits and risks.[3] The report, released in November 2003, said that medical studies on the hormone's effects in men age sixty-five and older are scant, short and inconclusive. Supposed benefits in such areas as strength, sexual function, mental acuity, and overall well-being have not been proven. Meanwhile, many doctors worry that the hormone could cause other problems, such as increasing the risk of prostate cancer and blood clots. The study, commissioned by the National Institutes of Health, stopped short of telling doctors to stop prescribing testosterone to older men whose levels, while lower than in youth, were not severely low or absent. In 2002, more than 1.75 million prescriptions for testosterone were written, a 170 percent increase from 1999, with the trend expected to continue. There are, indeed, cases of true deficiency—hypogonadism—and the Food and Drug Administration has approved the drug for this use. However, the majority of the prescriptions are written because of the supposed benefits and to try to counter the effects of aging.

Levels of all the sex hormones can be tested, but blood tests are not the most accurate method of testing. Because hormones circulate through the bloodstream attached to proteins and are not free-floating, a blood test will not pick up all the hormones that the body is producing. A saliva test is much more accurate, since it measures the free hormones as well.

HOW *NOT* TO NEED VIAGRA

Erectile dysfunction has been getting a lot of publicity lately, and when a brand-new drug, Viagra, hit the market in 1998, it zoomed immediately to the top of the list of best-selling drugs, helped by heavy advertising and lots of free samples. Impotence is one of the conditions that most men dread, and, unfortunately, most people don't know how to prevent or reverse it.

The most common cause of ED is lack of blood flow. Blood flow to the penis is dependent on enough testosterone (which most men have), a functioning neurological system (again, which most men have), and unhindered circulation. If the SAD diet can block arteries to the heart, brain, and all other parts of the body, it is not surprising that the same diet can block arteries to the entire genital region.

Scientists at the New England Research Institute found that fifty-two percent of men over forty have some degree of impotence, with the rate increasing significantly with age.[4] It was also found that these figures could be modified through changes in lifestyle. Stopping cigarette smoking is an obvious factor, but few realize that a change in diet can make a difference. The diet that reverses heart disease through cleaning out the arteries will have the same effect on the arteries that supply nutrients and oxygen to the genitalia.

In addition, the role of exercise seems to be much more important than previously realized. The Health Professionals Follow-up Study (HPFS) surveyed more than 51,000 male medical professionals, ages fifty-three to ninety, and asked them to rate their ability to perform sexually. They were also asked about important lifestyle habits such as smoking, drinking alcohol, and exercise. Exercise turned out to be the *most* significant factor in sexual performance, as those who exercised the most were one-third less likely to suffer from ED.[5]

EXERCISING YOUR KEGEL MUSCLES

We know that diet and exercise are extremely important, but most men have no idea that they need to exercise "down there." In a study that was done at the University of the West of England in Bristol, England, fifty-five men, with an average age of fifty-nine and suffering from ED for six months or longer, were given a protocol of Kegel exercises. They attended five weekly sessions and were given daily homework assignments. The results were that forty percent regained normal erectile function, with another thirty-five percent seeing improvement. These results, the researchers said, were the same results you'd expect to see in men taking Viagra for the same problem.[6]

According to Al Cooper, PhD, clinical director of the San Jose Marital and Sexuality Center, doing the Kegels on a regular basis will also produce more powerful orgasms.[7] Cooper explained that as men age, the pelvic muscles lose tone, there is less ejaculate formed, and therefore, orgasms get weaker. Doing the Kegels strengthens those muscles and thereby increases the intensity of orgasms. There is no reason why this wouldn't help women as well.

If you don't know what Kegels are, it's easy to learn. Next time you urinate, try stopping the flow of urine. Stop and start this process several times and, if you're successful, you will know you've got the right muscles. When you've learned control of those muscles, you can then control the muscles at any time and in any place. You could exercise them while sitting in a car at a stop light, or at your desk, or in bed.

Impotence needs to be treated promptly, because erections bring oxygen-rich blood to the penile blood vessels and nerves, and the longer between erections, the greater the damage to the lining of the blood vessels. Sufficient damage can eventually make erections impossible. The good news is that most ED is reversible by the diet and exercise program suggested here.

GETTING THE BODY YOU WANT

How about a nice flat tummy? What about nice, shapely thighs and calves? How about getting rid of those "love handles"? What about the flab that develops on the upper arms as you grow older? Women seem to be more concerned about stomachs, thighs, and arms, while men seem to be more concerned about that roll of fat that accumulates around the waist. Both men and women can have the bodies they desire if they're willing to do the work required.

In order to shape your body, you have to be smart about combining exercises effectively. For instance, you can do all the sit-ups in the world to remove that belly. However, if you've got excess fat in the abdominal area, all you're doing is building stronger muscles to move that fat up and down. Sit-ups alone won't do it, because there is no such thing as spot-reducing. If, however, you perform sit-ups coupled with a healthy vegan diet, you'll burn up the fat as well as build the muscles to support your abdomen.

The same is true with the thighs. Running, bicycling, squats, and lunges are all excellent exercises for building nice, strong muscles in the legs. But if you've got excess fat in the thighs, you're just building muscle *under* the fat on the thighs. With the diet we advocate, you'll also be burning up the fat that's covering those nice quadriceps. The same is true, of course, with the love handles. All the side bends in the world will not get rid of them, either. You need to run them off!

Despite the fact that all these exercises will not get rid of the fat on top of the muscles, I still recommend that you do them two or three times a week. Abdominal exercises are necessary to keep the stomach muscles strong, and bent-leg sit-ups (crunches) are among the most effective. Squats and lunges are very effective in keeping the thigh muscles strong and shapely. For strong, shapely arms, you should get a set of dumbbells of five or ten pounds and do bicep curls: Stand with your knees slightly bent, feet shoulder width apart, your spine in line (not swaybacked or hunched forward), and your hands by your sides; then, with a weight in each hand, raise the weights toward your chest, bending your elbows. Next, with feet and knees in the same position, bend forward from the waist so that your upper body is parallel to the floor and do tricep curls, where you straighten the arms behind you. For strong calves, ankles and feet, finish off with toe raises, standing on one leg and rising on tiptoe and back down. You should try for ten repetitions of each of these exercises and work up to three sets. This is a very basic routine; but it hits all the major body parts.

By exercising the muscles of the body parts you would like to improve, you will build more muscle and improve the shape to meet society's image of an attractive body, whether you're a man or a woman.

DEALING WITH VARICOSE VEINS

When I was a teenager, I started becoming aware of varicose veins in many, if not most, older women's legs. I noticed them in my mother and my aunt (my father's sister), whose varicose veins were so bad she had to have surgery to remove them. I remember thinking that that meant it was inevitable that I was going to get them as well since they were so present on both sides of the family. In fact, when I was eighteen, I noticed the first beginnings of spider veins on the backs of my legs. Fortunately for me, when I started daily running aged thirty-three, the veins disappeared. Now, at nearly seventy years of age, you can't find a single trace of varicose veins. I am therefore pretty well convinced that an exercise like running can prevent or even reverse varicose veins. This example is, of course, only anecdotal, and you'll be hard pressed to find a study proving that this works. Yet you've got nothing to lose and everything to gain by trying this.

FOR GUYS: IS BPH IN YOUR FUTURE?

BPH stands for Benign Prostatic Hypertrophy, and if you eat the SAD diet you are likely to get it. Urologists usually go on to say that if you live long enough, you'll also get cancer of the prostate. What we now know is that, in countries where they can't afford to eat the way we do, men are at a much lower risk for BPH or prostate cancer. The same diet that causes all these other diseases we've discussed can also cause an enlargement of the prostate and prostate cancer.

A frequent test of the prostate is a blood test known as the PSA, the prostate-specific antigen. The PSA measures the degree of disruption of the "architecture" of the prostate. In general, in evaluating the test, the lower the reading the better. A test called the DRE, the digital rectal exam, or even a recent ejaculation can cause a rise in the PSA, so test results are not always reliable. Elevated PSA counts do not necessarily mean cancer; conversely, a low reading does not necessarily mean one could not have cancer of the prostate. I am aware of a number of cases in which males over fifty have lowered their PSA counts simply by changing to a low-fat vegan diet. In any case, it is wise to be aware of the health of the prostate, since there are about 198,000 cases of prostate cancer diagnosed a year, and about 40,000 men die of that disease each year in this country.[8] In knowing all this, you will be one of only two percent of people in this country who are aware that there is a link between diet and prostate cancer.[9]

What is it that makes the difference between the high rates of prostate cancer in our country and the low rates in some other countries? Epidemiological studies show that men in countries with low-fat, low-animal-food diets have a lower risk of both BPH and prostate cancer, and that men who eat high-fat, high animal-food diets get these conditions—regardless of race or ethnicity.[10] Looking at the research, it is clear that diet is the major factor, and animal foods are implicated.

EXERCISE THAT MOST WILL LIKE

As stated earlier, we know that exercise is important for every part of the body, and that the genitalia are no exception. Erections, while not necessarily muscular in nature, have the same effect as exercise in that they increase the circulation of blood to the area. This serves to prevent damage to the lining of the arteries and to help keep the prostate healthy. It is safe to assume that the same holds true for women as well. Gynecologists also know that being sexually active helps maintain those parts and may prevent vaginal dryness and shrinkage. Now we know part of the reason why.

MENOPAUSE—THE SYMPTOMS
AND HOW TO AVOID THEM

Even though menopause is not a disease, it sure has a lot of women heading for their doctors to seek relief from hot flashes, weight gain, crying jags, irritability, insomnia, night sweats, vaginal dryness, and loss of libido. For more than fifty years, Premarin and other hormone replacement therapies have been prescribed as a solution. The estrogen in Premarin, the most widely used estrogen replacement drug, is derived from the urine of pregnant mares, who experience extreme cruelty, misery, and exploitation. Most of the foals born to these mares are killed because there is little use for them. Their mothers are kept continuously pregnant and tied up in cement-floored stalls just barely wide enough to accommodate them.[11] Desperate women who used the drug, however, didn't know and/or didn't care, because it relieved their symptoms, and doctors could count on having most of these patients for life. When research showed what had been suspected for years[12]—that it was too dangerous to allow women to continue using the drug—women felt they had been left in the lurch.

What few people have noticed is that women in developing countries don't suffer these symptoms. Their passage through menopause is celebrated, revered, and looked forward to. Why is there this difference?

DIET CAUSES MOST OF THE SYMPTOMS

We can rule out genetics, because Asian and African women don't have the symptoms of menopause unless and until they move to Western countries and start living the affluent lifestyle. Eating a diet high in rich animal foods changes the hormone levels of blood.

What we know now is that menopausal symptoms are caused not solely by a deficiency of estrogen, but most often by an *imbalance* of hormones, in other words, too much estrogen and not enough progesterone.[13] Diets that are high in fat cause an increase in estrogen through two different mechanisms: First, they lead to obesity, and a woman with more fat cells will produce and store more estrogen. Second, a high-fat diet is almost by definition a low-fiber diet, since fiber comes from plant foods, which are generally low in fat. With a low-fiber diet, the estrogen picked up by the liver for excretion through the bowel gets reabsorbed and re-circulated, and estrogen levels get too high. This increases a woman's risk of breast cancer. The progesterone is too low because when a woman stops ovulating (the definition of menopause), the corpus luteum of the egg stops producing progesterone. With no corpus luteum, there is no progesterone to balance the too-high estrogen. Therefore, with estrogen high and progesterone low, a dangerous hormonal imbalance occurs.

Eating a diet high in plant foods has the opposite effect. A woman's body continues to produce estrogen throughout her life, usually in a quantity sufficient to prevent menopausal symptoms. One may or may not want to add a plant source of progesterone.

If a woman's levels of estrogen are adequate and she still has menopausal symptoms, progesterone cream applied to the thinner skin of the inner arms, thighs, or abdomen will alleviate the symptoms in most cases. This cream also has the advantage of increasing bone density (up to forty percent in some cases) and increasing the body's sensitivity to thyroid hormone.[14] Some women who have been taking medications for both their bones and their thyroid have been able to get off both when starting the progesterone cream.

LACK OF EXERCISE

The other major difference between women in developing countries and ours is exercise—although poorer women don't call it "exercise"; they call it "work." Physical labor is the norm for most women in the world and, as a result, they don't get obese, their estrogen levels stay balanced, and they don't suffer from the symptoms of menopause that Western women do. In fact, in most poorer countries there is not even a translatable word for "hot flash." When you talk about "hot flashes" they don't understand and have trouble trying to imagine what you are talking about. They consider menopause a natural phase, something they look forward to, and an event that even earns them respect—very different from what women in this country expect.

HRT OR NOT HRT

In most cases, if the above recommended lifestyle changes are adopted, there is no need for hormone replacement therapy (HRT), which usually refers to a prescription for horse estrogen. As stated earlier, many Western women who used to take estrogen got cancer of the breast and cervix, again because of the imbalance of hormones. The drug companies came through with a "solution" to the problem. Instead of adding progesterone to their products (which they could have done but would have made no money, since no one can patent a natural substance), they made a synthetic form of progesterone, progestin, and were then able to charge a lot of money for their product. The major problem, however, was that there are a whole host of side effects from progestins. The major problems caused by taking HRT, besides breast and cervical cancer, include increased risk of cancer, strokes, blood clots, Alzheimer's,[15] hearing loss,[16] and asthma.[17]

All of this can be avoided by teaching women that a low-fat vegan diet coupled with daily, vigorous exercise will keep most, if not all, menopausal symptoms away. This plan may not make you popular with physicians or pharmaceutical companies, and that's why you are not seeing a big campaign for it. As in so many areas of healthy aging, you need to learn how to take care of yourself.

TOO MANY HYSTERECTOMIES[18]

Most women in this country have symptoms relating to either PMS or menopause. Problems such as heavy bleeding, painful cramps, fibroids, painful breasts, uterine prolapse, and enlarged uterus are due to a diet that is too high in animal products, which cause overstimulation of all the reproductive organs.

The typical medical response is to pull out the uterus and often the ovaries as well. However, women often don't realize how important the uterus is to their sexual response and anatomy— even after menopause, when the ovaries still produce hormones. A problem that may appear years later after a hysterectomy is incontinence, as the bladder and colon have lost their support. A much better solution is to change the diet to fruits and vegetables and get the correct hormone balance—and keep your uterus.

IS SOY THE ANSWER?

Much has been said in the media about soy products and their role as a phytoestrogen, meaning a plant source of estrogen. Another reason soy is heavily promoted is that people believe they need more protein and that soy is a good source of protein. The truth is that we don't really know. One side of the argument is that many soy products are refined, processed, and too high in fat. Some say that it's not good for men to get a lot of soy phytoestrogen. We know in Asia that soy has been safely consumed for centuries but only at moderate rates, so moderation is warranted if you include soy in your diet.

INCONTINENCE

Overactive bladder (OAB) is a common bladder control problem; however, it is not a normal part of aging. In fact, OAB is a common—and treatable—medical condition that is usually preventable and reversible.[19] Besides being embarrassing, OAB can affect your life. In a recent survey of OAB sufferers, many respondents reported that their condition disrupted their sleep, and more than half of them admitted to some degree of social withdrawal because of a fear of "accidents." About forty percent said that OAB negatively affected their enjoyment and frequency of sexual relationships.[20] You know you have OAB if you have to urinate every one to two hours during the day and at least twice at night, and you have strong, uncontrollable urges that you can't stop. You have "accidents" and "toilet-map," the latter meaning that you first find the bathrooms wherever you go before you do anything else. With OAB, the bladder contracts involuntarily, even when it is not full. The contraction causes several symptoms: a sudden urge to urinate, a constant sense of needing to urinate, and involuntary loss of urine due to an uncontrollable urge to urinate. This is called "urge incontinence."

OAB may be confused with other types of urinary problems such as "stress incontinence," when the muscles around the urethra (the tube that drains urine from the bladder) become weak and leakage occurs when coughing, sneezing, laughing, lifting, or exercising. "Overflow incontinence" occurs when your kidneys produce more urine than your bladder can hold, and the result is accidental loss of urine when a bathroom isn't nearby. These conditions can be helped by lifestyle changes such as doing more exercise, specifically the Kegels (which we covered earlier in this chapter), and avoiding caffeine, alcohol, and possibly very salty and spicy foods.

Urinary tract infections can be mistaken for OAB because they create the same sensation of constantly needing to urinate, coupled with an inability to pass more than a little at a time. A burning sensation while urinating is often a sign that you have a bacterial infection and not OAB. In men, benign prostatic hyperplasia (BPH) causes the enlarged prostate to put pressure on the urethra, which leads to incomplete emptying of the bladder and thus urinary frequency, urgency, and the need to urinate frequently during the night. The problem then is to deal with the prostate, which we covered earlier, and which can be kept healthy through a low-fat vegan diet.

Judging by the number of commercials and advertisements for adult diapers, incontinence is a major problem in this country. There are also all the drugs you see advertised accompanied by the jingle, "Gotta go, gotta go, gotta go right now!" As we age, all muscles will lose muscle tone if they are not properly exercised, and the pelvic floor muscles are no exception. Another complication of the SAD diet is that American women produce bigger babies, up to nine or ten pounds, and this can cause damage to the bladder and supporting structures. Women consuming a low-fat vegan diet produce healthy babies that at full term weigh six or seven pounds, which, according to Dr. John McDougall, is the normal weight for babies in the rest of the world and should be in the United States as well.[21]

CAUSES AND TREATMENTS

As mentioned earlier, hysterectomies may be responsible for some cases of incontinence, because of the loss of support for the bladder. With lack of exercise and ensuing weakness of the pelvic floor muscles, all the internal organs may start to sag, and this can lead to incontinence. A frequent treatment is the initiation of the Kegel exercises, discussed earlier. You should see improvement in bladder control in about six to twelve weeks.

In general, overall aerobic exercise such as running, walking, and swimming should help keep the pelvic floor muscles strong. Some women complain that they don't dare exercise because of the fear of an "accident." By ensuring an empty bladder at the start of exercise, they should be able to get through their exercise session safely. As they regain the strength of those muscles, the probability of an accident goes down. So here are more reasons to develop a program of daily vigorous exercise.

THE ROLE OF SELF-IMAGE
IN FEELING SENSUAL

In the exercise chapter we described a very basic exercise routine, which if done on a regular basis will help you feel good, look good, and even *be* good, which I define as being strong and lean. If you are all of these, you can't help but have a better self-image, and with a better self-image comes a feeling of being sensual. Nothing kills sensuality like being embarrassed or ashamed of your body, and following this diet and exercise program will give you a body to be very proud of. (Remember, also, that eating animal products leads to unpleasant smells. So, you'll smell great as well!)

BOTTOM LINE—WHAT WE KNOW FOR SURE

If you want to be a sexy senior for the rest of your life, eat a low-fat vegan diet and get daily, vigorous exercise. It'll relieve prostate problems for men, symptoms of menopause for women, and keep your bladder healthy. You'll look good, feel good, and, best of all, be good!

CHAPTER 15

ALZHEIMER'S, MAD COW DISEASE, CJD, AND MAINTAINING A SHARP MEMORY

ALZHEIMER'S: "THE HEALTH CARE CRISIS OF THE CENTURY"

According to a study published in August 2003 in the *Archives of Neurology*, as the Americans born between 1946 and 1964 creep toward their senior years, an Alzheimer's Disease (AD) epidemic of disturbing proportions is imminent.[1] It predicts that if no cure is found, Alzheimer's cases in the US will increase twenty-seven percent by 2020, seventy percent by 2030, and three hundred percent by 2050. The forecasts have led Sheldon Goldberg, president and chief executive of the Alzheimer's Association, to warn that the disease could destroy the health-care system and bankrupt Medicare and

Medicaid if left unchecked. Though several pharmaceutical companies are working on drugs they hope will improve memory and stop the Alzheimer's epidemic, a void exists in the meantime for those known as the "concerned well," boomers trying to hedge their bets against the disease and other memory loss.

There are also a host of small companies pitching dietary supplements such as ginkgo biloba, huperzine, and multivitamins. According to Patrick Rea, research director for the *Nutrition Business Journal*, US consumers spent $250 million in 2001 and $210 million in 2002 on supplements promoted as aids to mental acuity.[2] The supplements have not impressed most doctors and researchers enough to advocate their use. Experts say that instead of spending a lot of money on dietary supplements, boomers should consider mental exercises such as crossword puzzles, board games, reading, and other mental challenges. A twenty-one-year study published in June 2003 by doctors at Albert Einstein College of Medicine in New York reported that seniors who did crossword puzzles four days a week had a forty-seven percent lower risk of dementia than seniors who did puzzles once a week.[3]

DIET AND EXERCISE AND ALZHEIMER'S

It has been noted that people who don't get Alzheimer's are those with higher education, presumably because they are mentally more active. We know, however, that this is not the only factor, because one study reported that meat-eaters experienced Alzheimer's or some form of dementia at three times the rate of vegetarians.[4] High blood levels of homocysteine (greater than 15 micromoles per liter) have been identified as a risk factor for Alzheimer's and dementia.[5] In fact, the higher the homocysteine, the higher the risk. In one study, homocysteine levels decreased by up to twenty percent in subjects just one week after switching to a vegan diet.[6] More evidence that diet is a factor is that the risk of getting Alzheimer's is five times higher in the US than it is in China or Nigeria,[7] where the diets are less meat- and dairy-based.

Exercise also helps. Researchers at the University of Washington took 153 Alzheimer's patients and gave half of them thirty minutes of daily exercise. The other patients acted as a control group, and both groups got "routine" care. After two years, the exercise group was still active, had less depression, and was in much better physical shape, with fewer signs of frailty.[8] In another study done at Utah State University, four hundred women, aged seventy to eighty, were followed for eighteen years. Their Body Mass Index (BMI) and results of neuropsychiatric tests were followed. On average, the women who developed Alzheimer's had a BMI two to three points higher than the mentally healthy women. At age seventy, each 1.0 increase in BMI raised Alzheimer's risk by thirty-six percent. This is highly significant because of the increasing obesity in the US and other Western countries. With the present estimates of 22 million people with Alzheimer's by the year 2025, the numbers will be even higher when current trends toward greater numbers of obese people are factored in.[9]

There is much research going on to figure out how our brains work. Until then, we are not fully certain as to how to prevent or reverse many of the brain diseases of the aging. One very exciting discovery reported by John J. Ratey, MD, author of *A User's Guide to the Brain*, is that the brain *can* produce new brain cells. It has long been taught that you only get what you're born with, and that alcohol, for example, destroys brain cells that can never be replaced. Fortunately, the brain does recover and can maintain its sharpness as it ages.

We know that aerobic exercise improves mood by increasing levels of dopamine and serotonin to the brain. It has been found that attention and learning are also improved with higher levels of these hormones. Just as exercise can enable the body to create corollary circulation (the heart's own bypass), the brain can do the same thing. Vigorous exercise increases the circulation to the brain as well as to the rest of the body.

We also now know that keeping the brain active and challenged is extremely important as we age. We should keep looking for new ways to do old things—such as holding the toothbrush with our left hand if we're right-handed, learning a new language, taking music lessons, etc. Dance lessons and Tai Chi are doubly beneficial because, besides the learning that takes place, these practices also help increase social skills. Studies have also shown that physically fit older people do just as well on mental tests as younger people. Being passionate about something is also important, as it provides the motivation to strive and to learn. It also creates a much more satisfying life.

Any form of aerobic exercise is good. Aerobic exercise causes the release of Brain-Derived Neurotrophic Factor (BDNF), which acts as a "fertilizer" and appears to promote the growth of new cells and strengthen existing connections.[10] This enables more learning and allows memory to stay active.

MENTAL FITNESS

How often have you walked into a room and then wondered what you came to get, or opened the refrigerator and forgot whether you were putting something in or taking something out? As we age, memory lapses can make us fear that we're losing our mental sharpness. However, since we know we can add neurons no matter how old we are, just how do we keep sharp? Along with Senior Fitness, we need Mental Fitness.

Each neuron in the brain has branches called *dendrites*, and whenever the brain is stimulated by a new experience, new dendrites form. Here are five exercises to do along with your physical exercises:

- Use your non-dominant hand in your everyday activities. We've already given the example of brushing your teeth holding the toothbrush with your other hand. Try writing with your left hand if you're right-handed. This will help develop your speech abilities in the non-dominant side of the brain as well.
- "Lose" one of your five senses. We already know that blind people develop their other senses to a much higher level than those who have their sight. Put on a blindfold and try dressing yourself. Put in earplugs and see how well you do with lip-reading. Deprive yourself of smell by holding your nose and try to identify different tastes of food. These activities will help you develop different neural pathways.
- Change your routine. If you always take the elevator, take the stairs. Rearrange the dishes in the kitchen. Wear your watch on the opposite wrist. Run backwards. Even small changes activate the cortex and hippocampus, the part of the brain crucial for memory formation.
- Get a new hobby. If you're not computer literate, now's the time to get started. You can also learn a foreign language, or take up oil painting. Try learning Braille or American Sign Language. Complex skills activate the nonverbal and emotional centers in the cortex of the brain.
- Get more social. Interaction with others can be one of the best brain exercises because it brings all the senses into play. It forces you to think quickly and hones your speaking skills. For example, start a book club or an exercise group, or arrange a vegan potluck.

THE ROLE OF DIET IN BRAIN HEALTH

The US Department of Agriculture has published studies showing that blueberries rank near the top in antioxidants among forty different fruits and vegetables.[11] A number of other studies have shown that blueberries boost brain power and restore memory, coordination, and balance lost with age. The *APA Monitor* in December 2001 reported a study that showed that dark colored fruits and vegetables and physical exercise reduced cognitive decline in older people. Memory improved significantly at both the statistical and functional level—and change was most dramatic in those who ate blueberries, from a half a cup to a cup daily.

MAD COW DISEASE AND CJD

Mad Cow Disease, or bovine spongiform encephalopathy (BSE), is a disease of cattle that attacks the nervous system. It was first recognized in England in 1986 and in the form of variant Creutzfeldt-Jacob disease (vCJD) has caused the deaths of more than 100 people who had eaten beef infected with BSE. It has been spreading slowly ever since. Switzerland discovered BSE in its cattle and along with England has noted an increase in CJD cases. No one knows what exactly causes the classic form of CJD, but there's evidence to suggest that it may be caused by the consumption of infected meat as well. Scientists believe these diseases are caused by prions, self-replicating proteins found in brain and nerve tissue that are almost impossible to destroy by known methods of sterilization, heat, chemicals, etc. The condition in both cows and humans is an always-fatal brain disease that causes microscopic, sponge-like holes in the brain and has also been found in sheep, elk, and mink. The symptoms are memory loss, difficulty keeping one's balance and walking, an inability to talk and swallow, and, finally, death.

This is an area of great concern for many scientists and economists because of the devastating nature of this disease.[12] First, it is difficult to diagnose because there are no specific tests that can determine whether a living person has CJD, Alzheimer's Disease, or another type of dementia. It is only when an autopsy is performed that the presence of the disease can be known. Several studies have found that autopsies reveal three to thirteen percent of patients diagnosed with Alzheimer's or dementia actually suffered from CJD.[13] These numbers may sound low, but there are four million Alzheimer's cases and hundreds of thousands of cases of dementia in the US. Three to thirteen percent of those cases could add up to thousands more CJD cases going undetected. Complicating this is the fact that fewer autopsies are being performed. Although autopsies used to be performed on approximately half of all cases of dementia, the frequency has dropped to fifteen percent or less in the US. The National Center for Health Statistics, a branch of the Centers for Disease Control, stopped collecting autopsy data in 1995.

While autopsies have been declining, the number of deaths attributed to Alzheimer's has increased more than fifty-fold since 1970, going from 857 deaths then to nearly 50,000 in 2000. Though it is unlikely that the dramatic increase in Alzheimer's is due entirely to undiagnosed CJD cases, it could explain some of the increase, according to Laura Manueldis, Section Chief of Surgery in the Neuropathology Department at Yale University, who conducted a 1989 study that found thirteen percent of Alzheimer's patients actually suffered from CJD.[14]

With the discovery of Mad Cow Disease in both the US and Canada, it is obvious that the most prudent response is to avoid eating cows—just more evidence of the risks that come with eat-

ing animals as food. In the case of Mad Cow Disease, even consuming beef extract, beef stock, and beef flavoring puts you at risk.

BOTTOM LINE—WHAT WE KNOW FOR SURE

To lower your risk of getting Alzheimer's, Mad Cow Disease,
Creutzfeldt-Jacob Disease, and memory loss, eat a low-fat vegan
diet and get daily, vigorous exercise.

CHAPTER 16

KEEPING YOUR SENSES

GROWING OLDER SEEMS to mean the gradual loss of many of our senses. This can be disastrous because the dimming of our senses gradually cuts us off from both our physical and social environment and makes us more vulnerable to a number of risks, including accidents and social isolation. No one is quite certain to what extent a good diet and exercise program can delay the onset of the loss; however, we do know that maintaining an antioxidant-rich blood supply to the eyes, ears, organs of proprioception (which help us maintain balance), teeth and gums will give us the best chance of holding on to these capabilities as long as possible.

VISION

Most people rely on vision more than any other of the senses, because so much of the information about our environment comes through our eyes. Unfortunately, loss or degradation of vision is all too frequent among people as they age. Cataracts, glaucoma, and macular degeneration are the three most common causes of vision impairment. Cataracts are thought to be inevitable as we age; however, we know that smokers (nicotine causes impaired circulation) and people who consume dairy products are more prone to have them. Studies have also shown that it is possible to prevent these conditions, or at least stop the progression, by adopting the lifestyle patterns advocated in this book.[1] While it may be impossible to prevent some loss as we age, there are things we can do to give ourselves the best chance for good vision for the rest of our lives.

In a recent study, people with glaucoma who exercised regularly for three months reduced their interocular pressure (IOP) an average of twenty percent. These people rode stationary bikes four times per week for forty minutes. Doctors saw measurable improvements in eye pressure and physical conditioning at the end of three months. These beneficial effects were maintained by continuing to exercise at least three times per week, and lowered IOP was lost if exercise was stopped for more than two weeks.[2]

According to William Harris, MD, the incidence of Age Related Macular Degeneration (ARMD) appears to have increased over the past fifty years.[3] He claims that it was not a common problem when he was in medical training forty years ago and that his 1983 edition of a text on general ophthalmology barely mentions it. It's a different story today. The loss of vision occurs when the growth of abnormal blood vessels seeps under the macula, the central part of the retina. The vessels then leak fluid, causing scar tissue that destroys central vision. This is known as the "wet" form of ARMD and is the leading cause of blindness in the US, with 200,000 new cases each year. Dr. Harris believes that low intake of beta-carotene, Vitamin C and E, as well as lutein and zeaxanthin, is responsible. Leafy greens are excellent sources of all these nutrients.

The eyes rely on our circulatory system for nutrition, oxygen, and the transporting of waste products. We also know that people who have diabetes and arteriosclerosis are at greater risk for eye problems. Since we know that eating the SAD diet leads to diabetes and arteriosclerosis, it is logical to assume that the SAD diet also contributes to cataracts, glaucoma, and macular degeneration. Therefore, it makes good sense for us to eat a healthy vegan diet (which provides the nutrients) and to get daily effective exercise (to increase the circulation as much as possible to all parts of the eyes). While the beta-carotene in carrots has long been recognized as important in vision, it has also been recognized that leafy greens are important in providing the nutrients that the eyes need most. For me, this information was so important that I started adding leafy greens to my breakfast. After all, I reasoned, why not get those nutrients circulating in my bloodstream as early as possible in the day? In addition, it just makes good sense to protect the eyes from ultraviolet radiation from the sun, so be sure to wear good sunglasses whenever you are outdoors.

HEARING

Another loss that senior folks frequently notice is in their ability to hear. The ear has tiny bones, the ossicles, which vibrate according to sound waves, transmitting sound from the eardrum. When they can't vibrate, they can't conduct sound. There are also the cilia, tiny hairs in fluid in the cochlea that play a role in the conduction of sound, especially the high-pitched sounds. These are lost as we age. We also know that smokers are more prone to losing their hearing for the same reason as they lose their sight (and virtually everything else). Here again, it just makes good sense that the delicate parts of the ear with their tiny blood vessels need to have good circulation. If the arteries and capillaries are not clogged with plaque—in other words, if we are eating high-nutrient foods and exercising daily to keep the circulation going—we have our best chance to keep our hearing intact.

According to Robert Anderson, MD, president and acting executive director of the American Board of Holistic Medicine, partial hearing loss can often be reversed by eliminating dairy products from our diet.[4] John McDougall, MD, would agree.[5] Anecdotal evidence has shown that patients who stop consuming dairy products and foods rich in whey (such as some breads and pastries) have experienced significant improvements in hearing tests. Anderson and McDougall's theory is that age-related hearing loss could be caused by an allergic response to the protein in dairy. It is also possible that *any* animal protein could cause the same reaction.

What you should never do is expose your ears to animal proteins or to loud noises. An example of what could be achieved if we protected our ears from both of these is the Masaan, an isolated pastoral tribe in and around Sudan. Auditory studies have shown that the Masaan lose only a quarter as much of their sensitivity at all frequencies at all ages as Westerners.[6] Because they rarely encounter loud noises and do not have the diseases we do, such as heart disease and high blood pressure, it is a reasonable supposition that both diet and noise play an important role in maintaining good hearing.

KEEPING YOUR BALANCE

One of the problems people notice as they age is that they tend to lose their balance more frequently. Obviously, being unable to keep your balance means that you're more likely to fall, which could lead to devastating injuries such as a broken hip, wrist or leg. An astonishing twelve million older Americans fall each year, resulting in about ten thousand deaths.[7] Falling is also the *main* cause of accidental death in people over the age of sixty-five. The good news is that balance is a skill that can be trained and improved. In fact, it *must* be, or else, like all our other skills, we will lose the ability. Balancing exercises are really a coordination exercise between the brain, your nerves and spinal cord, and your muscles. Here are two very simple balance exercises that you can do at home.

1. Standing, lift your right knee out in front of you and raise your arms out to the side like the wings of a bird. Hold this position for at least thirty seconds and then repeat with the left leg. Repeat each of these positions several times a day. Then try closing your eyes while you do it.
2. Standing, lift your right leg out to the side and hold it out for at least thirty seconds, again with both arms out to the side. Next, do the same with the left leg out to the side. Repeat this also several times a day, and then with eyes closed.

If you are especially unstable, be sure to have a wall, a sturdy piece of furniture, or even another person close by, to grab in case you need additional support.

Balancing exercises are the most effective means to help prevent falls. Other suggestions are Tai Chi classes, physical therapy lessons, and fall-prevention exercise classes offered by some community fitness centers. It is also possible to have an occupational therapist check your home for fall hazards by contacting the American Occupational Therapy Association (301-652-2682, www.aota.org).

DENTAL CARE

People rarely think about their teeth in terms of diet and exercise. However, both play a role in keeping strong, healthy teeth. It makes sense that if your teeth, gums, and the bones that hold the teeth in place are getting all the nutrients they need and none of the harmful substances in animal foods and tobacco, you will have a much healthier mouth. This seems to be the case, according to Dr. Lia Dominici-Bly, a practicing dentist in Honolulu, Hawaii. She is a firm believer in a good diet, flossing after every meal, and in brushing effectively with a manual toothbrush or power brushes, such as the Sonicare and Braun brands. I brush for one whole minute for each quadrant. Another form of oral exercise is chewing. Since I eat my fruits and vegetables primarily raw, my jawbones have remained very strong. One of the drawbacks of juicing is that you're depriving your teeth, gums and bones of valuable exercise.

One of the problems that aging may bring is dingy, darkened teeth. Aging baby boomers have become more focused on treating their teeth with whitening products. While this does not deal directly with senior fitness, I think we all feel and look healthier with nice, white teeth in a nice, broad smile. There are home kits, tooth-whitening centers, and procedures performed by dentists. Teeth can be turned snowy white by the application of hydrogen peroxide and carbamide peroxide. These substances may be applied in trays that are fitted to the teeth or in strips; when done properly, this does not harm the your teeth or gums. After whitening is completed, there may be a gradual relapse back to the original color. Touch-ups may be necessary to prevent a relapse from occurring at all.

BOTTOM LINE—WHAT WE KNOW FOR SURE

To keep your vision, hearing, balance, and teeth, eat a low-fat, whole-food vegan diet and get daily, vigorous exercise. Much of what we formerly thought was inevitable loss of our senses due to aging we now know is caused by damage done to our eyes, ears, and teeth—and is therefore preventable.

CHAPTER 17

Motivation—How to Get It, How to Keep It

MOTIVATION IS VITALLY important for senior fitness. The first thing you need is a goal—a goal that will ensure you won't quit your fitness program. Here are three tips that can help you succeed.

1. If your goal is to be a fit, healthy person, develop a clear picture of what that would look like in you—for example, looking lean, mean, trim, and strong. Be much more specific than something vague such as "lose some weight" or "improve health."
2. Emphasize the positive. List the rewards that are most meaningful to you, such as having more energy, feeling fantastic, needing no medications, being able to travel the world, etc.
3. Make specific plans. Make a date with yourself. Get a monthly calendar and write down specific appointments. For example, write down "weights" at eight A.M. three times a week, Monday, Wednesday, and Friday. Your goals need to be specif-

ic, measurable, attainable. Have a deadline, and make it something you can write out, such as "Run a 5K race by next June." Write this down and post it on your refrigerator or in your clothes closet where you can see it on a regular basis to remind you of what you need to do to get ready. It's even better if you can get one or more others to share your goal, as group support is always helpful if and when you start having second thoughts about your goal. It's also useful to have a timeline so that you can post your progress at, say, one week, one month, two months, etc.

POSITIVE REINFORCEMENT

One of the first principles of psychology that I learned in college was that we tend to do that which is positively reinforced (rewarded), and we tend to avoid that which is either punished or not reinforced. This is called a "conditioned response." Think of the example of a child touching a hot stove and being immediately conditioned not to touch the stove again. In Pavlov's famous experiments, he rang a bell just before feeding his dogs. The food caused the dogs to salivate, but after a few trials, the bell itself would cause the dogs to salivate, an obviously conditioned response.

Most of our adult behavior is not quite so simple, but the principles still apply. For example, I ran a race this morning. When my alarm went off at 5:30 A.M., I was conditioned to get out of bed to get ready for the race. During the race itself, I pushed to try to get a faster time, which was very uncomfortable, but I thought about my finish time and the fact that the race would soon be over. Sure enough, crossing the finish line, I had a great big smile on my face, and at the award ceremony I collected a gold medal. You can bet that I was very positively reinforced, not only at the finish line and at the award ceremony, but also to get out there and train harder at my next speed-training session. I also have a lot of fun at these races, which turns out to be another way of positively reinforcing my exercise program.

SEE RESULTS WITHIN HOURS

Yesterday I heard a doctor on a talk-radio show telling listeners that they could avoid taking cholesterol-lowering drugs just by changing their diet. My ears perked up—finally, I thought, the word was getting out and we were making some progress. But then the doctor said that it would take three or four months to see results. I almost screamed at the radio, because I have repeatedly seen real drops in cholesterol within two *weeks*! My own cholesterol went from 236 to 160 in three weeks, and I'm convinced that if it had been tested sooner it would have shown the results sooner. In any case, that much of a drop in two or three weeks shows how quickly our bodies respond to effective dietary change.

You would actually see changes within two hours if you could look in the backs of your eyeballs! After a high-fat meal, the blood vessels are bulging, twisted and ropey, and the red blood cells sticky and sludgy. (It's two hours after a high-fat meal that one is at highest risk of a heart attack or stroke.) After a low-fat meal, the blood vessels are smooth and straight, with no stickiness or sludge. It's too bad that we can never know of all the heart attacks and strokes that are *avoided* by not eating the wrong foods. If we could only point out those people who had avoided that heart attack or stroke, there'd be a lot more people paying attention to what we're saying. Results can be faster than most people think.

AT-HOME TESTING—KNOWLEDGE IS POWER

A major problem in making healthful changes is that feedback is not always as immediate as looking at the backs of your eyeballs. If you knew that, after every steak or hamburger, the person eating it keeled over and died, you would have a strong disincentive to eat meat. The problem is that, in most cases, you don't see the harmful effects of a poor diet for years. The same is true for all the other degenerative diseases we've discussed in this book.

One way to get feedback on the effectiveness of your changes to a healthier lifestyle is to have some at-home tests. Probably the most common home test involves the *bathroom scales*. This is a very rough guide to how much body fat you are carrying, and whether or not you are putting more on or taking some off. There are now bathroom scales that also estimate your percentage of body fat directly. This is more likely what you are interested in— how much of your body weight is actually fat.

Another common home test is a *thermometer* for measuring body temperature. A fever is a clue that the body is fighting some kind of infection. A body temperature that is too low could indicate an underactive thyroid. Be sure to check what your "normal" is, because it can vary from 97 to 99 degrees Fahrenheit.

A *blood pressure kit* is also a good test to have at home. Elevated blood pressure is a sure sign of encroaching ailments and a warning to make a lifestyle change. The loss of just a few pounds in weight can lower blood pressure significantly. Or, if you're already at a normal weight, you can see your blood pressure drop by not eating refined, processed foods and starting a running program. Alcohol can also increase blood pressure. An at-home kit to track blood pressure is frequently a superior method to going to the doctor's office because of the prevalence of "white coat hypertension," where blood pressure goes up because of the stress of being in the doctor's office. Keep a log so that you don't rely on memory, and test it several times a day until you see a pattern. You'll also have to be sure the blood pressure kit is accurate by having it calibrated annually.

Drug stores and pharmacies carry a number of different kinds of test kits. I bought the test for *glucose* (blood sugar) and found it fascinating to see how my body reacted during these tests. For example, within minutes of eating, my blood sugar started rising. This is good if you're starting out on a run or any other exercise. You can also test for your *total serum cholesterol.* When switching from the SAD diet to the vegan diet, it can be pretty exciting to watch your cholesterol drop like the proverbial rock.

There is the fecal occult (which means not visible to the naked eye) blood test kit for colon cancer. The simplest one involves dropping a piece of treated tissue into the toilet after a bowel movement. A color change indicates the presence of blood, an early sign of possible cancer of the colon and the need for further testing by a physician. You do need to prepare for this test by being sure not to eat meat for the day or two before the test, lest you end up positive for someone else's blood.

Current testing for osteoporosis involves exposure to radiation. It is neither convenient nor cheap. You can, however, do your own at-home osteoporosis test by very accurately measuring your *height.* Osteoporosis entails loss of bone mass, and in your spine you've got twenty-four separate bones. If each one of these bones, the vertebrae, loses just a tiny fraction of bone, that loss is soon apparent in loss of height. Use a carpenter's square, or a book if you don't have a carpenter's square, and put it on your head, taking care to get an exact ninety-degree angle as you stand up straight against a wall. Have someone make a mark on the wall, noting the height. Walk away, turn around, do it again, walk away, and do it once more, then take an average of the three readings. You want to get as accurate a measure as possible. Another caution: Be sure to measure yourself at the same time of day, because you may be as much as an inch taller first thing in the morning, losing that inch throughout the day.

Below is the *Amsler grid to test for macular degeneration*, a simple piece of paper with a crosshatch of lines. Test each eye separately. The lines should appear straight, but are wavy if you have macular degeneration. I've added an example here so you can take the test right now.

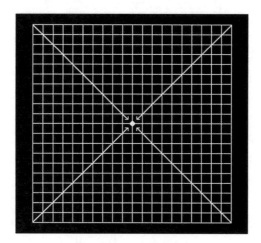

The Amsler Grid

There are also *saliva tests for estrogen, progesterone and testosterone* levels. These tests are more accurate than the blood tests done at the laboratory, because blood tests only measure the free hormones and most hormones are bound to proteins.

You could even do home *urine tests* to measure *pH* (acidity level), *sugar* (to test for diabetes) or *menopause* (by testing for higher than normal levels of FSH, the follicle-stimulating hormone). There are also urine test strips that will change color when a urinary tract infection is present. Obtain these tests by getting the appropriate strips from a pharmacy or lab. A very simple test for *dehydration* consists of looking at the color of your urine. While this test is not completely reliable, a dark yellow indicates a concentration level that probably means you're not drinking enough water. Constant monitoring will give you an indication of what your normal range of color is.

When I asked Dr. William Harris once whether or not I should have a particular diagnostic test, his response was, "You can never know too much about your body." That guidance has been extremely useful, and I have applied it ever since. This is why I started collecting all these home tests so I can know as much as possible "what condition my condition is in."

BEING YOUR OWN COACH

You're probably well aware of the fact that as you go through life you are subject to other people's opinions about what you should and should not do about any number of things. There are the ultra-conservatives who think that you should never take risks. On the other hand, there are those reckless types who dive into challenges without thinking through a plan to succeed. An example of the former is a running friend who was discouraged from entering a marathon by her parents because she "might get hurt." An example of the latter would be, "You're not trained for this marathon, but I'm sure that you can get through the 26.2 miles— one way or another!" With any luck you are somewhere in the middle—and that's why you will have to be your own coach.

Your inner "coach" needs to say to you, "Yes, you're a good runner, but let's plan for the next marathon and start a marathon training program now." Once you start the training program, you will be tempted to quit. These will be times when you have to assess what you are doing and why, and to have a plan. This is where having the running journal that I talked about earlier becomes more important. Journals have the power to motivate as they give objective feedback on your progress. You have to picture yourself crossing that finish line and imagine how you will feel when you've accomplished a major goal. That's when you go back to work and follow the plan of the training program. Most often, I have found that we don't aim high enough!

OVERCOMING "CHALLENGES"

In April 1998, I was on my bike training for another triathlon when a truck carrying a load of kitchen cabinets made a sudden left turn as the driver realized that he had almost passed the street where he was to make his delivery. Unfortunately for me, I was coming from the opposite direction and happened to be in the middle of the intersection, and he plowed right into me. I saw the truck coming but could not get out of its way, and the impact sent me flying through the air. When I landed, I was in excruciating pain. I looked down at my left leg and saw a number of bumps that turned out to be broken bones. The mere raising of my head caused extreme pain in my right hip. My first thought was, "How am I ever going to do that triathlon in three months?"

A driver in another vehicle stopped and yelled that he was calling 911. An ambulance was there within minutes and I got a very fast ride to the emergency room. The injuries were devastating. X-rays and an MRI showed that my left leg had been shattered where the truck's bumper had hit me, and I had three cracks in my right pelvis where I had landed after being thrown into the air. As bad as I thought these injuries were, the doctors in the ER marveled at the fact that I was still alive. They said that if I had not been as fit as I was, I would probably have been killed, and that I should consider myself "lucky to be alive."

As I worked through months of a long, very painful recovery, trying to get back to running, an orthopedist said, "You need to *face facts*, that you will never be able to run again, much less race." The orthopedist's words immediately brought to mind my diagnosis with breast cancer, where I was told I might not have much longer to live. My response then had been to change to a vegan diet and do the Ironman Triathlon. My response to this new pro-nouncement was to double my physical therapy (PT). My med-ical insurance covered PT twice a week, so I added two more ses-sions of therapy a week and paid for it myself.

Even though I had to miss the triathlon I had been training for, the investment in intense exercise still paid off handsomely. I knew there was no way I was going to be off my crutches in time to enter any of the track events in the upcoming Senior Olympics, so the next best thing for me to do was to volunteer to be a timer. As I watched each of the different events, I got an idea. I could surely run the 100-meter dash on crutches! The race director and President of our Hawaii Senior Olympics, Mark Zeug, thought I was crazy but supported my decision. Sure enough, I toed the start line along with all the able-bodied ath-letes, and when the gun went off I took off as fast as I could—on my crutches. Of course, I had a *very* slow time, but I made it—and, since I was the only one in my sixty-five-to-sixty-nine age group, I won another gold medal!

My recovery accelerated as I continued to get as much exer-cise as I could, and I looked forward to being able to race a "real" race. Four months later I felt that I was recovered enough to enter the Squamish 10K in British Columbia, where I happened to be traveling at the time. I entered and, incredibly, again won an age-group first place in my first race just four months after that near-fatal truck accident.

Since my race times were considerably slower than before the truck hit me, I started to focus on speed work. I had run down to Ala Moana Beach Park, one of my favorite running courses, and coming toward me was a strong, young male runner looking like a gazelle. Inspired to emulate him, I immediately picked up my speed, tripped on a raised crack in the sidewalk, and went flying! I landed full force on my right shoulder. Another trip to the Emergency Room.

"No more running for you, young lady!" Those were the

words out of the mouth of the ER doctor as he walked in with my x-rays. I couldn't believe what he was saying and confusedly said, "Why? What do you mean?" He shoved the x-ray under the lighted box and said, "You can *not* afford any more injuries like this!" He pointed at the bones of my shoulder and what I saw made me sick. The head of the humerus, the upper arm bone, was shattered. As the doctor was putting me in a sling, he said, "It's going to take six to eight weeks to heal—if you're lucky, considering your age" (I was sixty-five at the time).

Well, I had been through this before. I knew that being extremely fit already, continuing to eat my low-fat vegan diet, and pushing the physical therapy, I would heal in half the predicted time. Sure enough, an x-ray taken at three weeks showed the bones knitting nicely and I was cleared to start swimming again. I was, of course, already back to running.

GIVING BACK

I have already mentioned that while I was still on crutches and theoretically couldn't race, I volunteered to be a timer. I've been president of both my running clubs, race director for several races, coach for budding triathletes, and have written a number of articles and two books on running, nutrition, and fitness. In each of these instances, I've been amply rewarded. In the first case, that of being a timer at the Senior Olympics, the reward was simply being there at the start line when I thought racing was impossible. That was when it dawned on me I could do the race on crutches. Through all of the other activities, I met people I wouldn't have otherwise encountered and learned a lot about race administration and coaching. While writing articles and books, I've been forced to do research, organize, and put thoughts in order, which has been a great benefit to me as well as, I hope, to my readers. By volunteering my time, I've always been very amply rewarded.

REFRAMING

The process of "reframing" is a powerful and productive technique. It consists of taking your evaluation of a situation and turning it around so that you end up with a more objective and positive evaluation.

For example, I recall reading a story of an old farmer who had an only son who happened to be born with a clubfoot. The farmer had thought ever since his son's birth that life was unfair to both of them. Then came a call to war and all the other young men in the surrounding area were called to fight. Because he had a clubfoot, the farmer's son had been excused. When all the soldiers from his town were killed in action, the farmer realized that his son's medical condition had saved his life.

Another example of reframing might be if your elderly mother is still driving her car, and after three fender benders and failing eyesight you suggest she stop driving. Her reaction is swift and negative. You then realize that her driving is not really the issue—but her independence is. Once the problem is reframed, you can help her look at alternatives such as the bus, a taxi, or a car service paid for by the proceeds from the sale of her car.

Think of the worst possible scenario of things that can go wrong in life. Then look for the advantages that lie therein, because they are usually there—somewhere. You've probably heard the story about the boy who, when confronted with a room full of manure, said excitedly, "There has to be a pony in here somewhere!" The process of reframing can help in most situations in life, and it is helpful to practice the technique frequently so that when an emotional crisis comes up, you're already adept at reframing.

OTHER CHALLENGES—ADDICTIONS

For some, addictions can be a real problem. Whether smoking, drinking alcohol, taking other drugs, eating animal foods, or overeating, the use of these substances to satisfy some psychological need becomes a deeply ingrained habit that many find very difficult to give up. Even if you have tried and failed to give up a bad habit, you should keep trying. For many, substitution works, and the best substitute is exercise. When the urge for a cigarette or a drink hits, head out the door for a walk or a run. It is the same with overeating. If you were to apply this technique for twenty-one days, you would theoretically have broken the habit and replaced it with one that will do you far more good.

BOTTOM LINE—WHAT WE KNOW FOR SURE

By eating a low-fat vegan diet and getting daily vigorous exercise, you will realize that you have control over your health, and that should provide all the motivation you need. You will never again want to compromise your health.

CHAPTER 18

PUTTING IT ALL TOGETHER

D ID YOU HAPPEN to notice that at the end of each
chapter, the Bottom Line got to be pretty boring and
repetitious? Yes, as someone once said to me, "Oh, you
always give the same answer for every health problem—change
your diet and start exercising."

Well, it's true. Eating the Standard American Diet causes what
some are calling the "*grand disease*"—in other words, a single disease with a size, scope, and extent never before seen. The symptoms of this condition are heart disease, cancer, stroke, diabetes,
arthritis, hypertension, osteoporosis, obesity, and so on. To cure
oneself of this new disease, one has to get rid of the cause—the
SAD diet.

Exercise is also important because of a rule of physiology I
have invoked throughout this book: "Use it or lose it." It is simply
true that the fit person is likely to live longer than the unfit person. A case in point: The Cooper Clinic in Dallas, Texas has done
much research on fitness. In 1989, it published the first report
from the Aerobic Center Longitudinal Study on the relationship
of fitness to mortality. The results indicated that unfit men and

women were much more likely to die than those who were even moderately fit. This study has been cited nearly a thousand times in other scientific publications, and is one of the most influential studies on exercise published in the past twenty years. It was used as one of the key pieces of evidence to support public health recommendations for increasing physical activity issued by the US Surgeon General, National Institutes of Health, Centers for Disease Control and Prevention, and the American Heart Association.[1]

In another study that reached the same conclusion, the Cooper Clinic also showed that unfit men who begin to exercise and improve their low level of fitness can cut their risk of dying by fifty percent.[2]

Of course, there are other diseases that affect seniors that I have not covered in this book because they are less common. However, there's an old saying among diagnosticians: When you hear hooves—think horses, not zebras. This means that when presented with a problem, look first for the most common diagnosis, not some rare exotic entity. And that is what I have done here. I am not trying to diagnose anyone's problems, and your personal physician is the first one to go to when you have a medical problem. However, keep in mind that diet and exercise are extremely powerful in maintaining and regaining health.

Science is always adding new discoveries from all the studies that are currently going on, and it is impossible to have a book that is completely up to date on all the latest findings. Most of the studies, however, revolve around finding new ways to diagnose or treat disease. For example, scientists are perfecting a new technique to find breast cancer at a stage earlier than a mammogram does. This, of course, does nothing to *prevent* the breast cancer from starting in the first place. What this book advocates is a lifestyle that *prevents* disease, and I for one don't believe there are going to be too many more new discoveries better than what we know already. It is up to you to determine whether you feel that I have presented the best possible diet and exercise program.

I want to emphasize for the final time that what I have presented in this book is more than just a diet and exercise program. I also want to stress that it is not an "all or nothing" situation. *Any* improvement in your diet will help you, as will *any* increase in how often and how intensely you exercise. However, whether you like it or not, what you eat and whether you move your body, and how often, form the base of the health pyramid on top of which everything else about your health is built. I cannot emphasize enough how precious health is; once you lose your health, you've lost almost everything. If we have good health, then everything else is merely frosting on the cake.

HAVING AND BEING A FRIEND

As we age, we find that social relationships change. Our preferences in people change, our interests change, and we're always gaining new perspectives. What doesn't change is that we still need social structure. People with a good social support system live longer and healthier lives than those who don't. To make sure we keep our friends, we first need to *be* a friend, and this includes maintaining an interest in others beside ourselves. Most people, as they age, find their concerns turning to their own health, and the old stereotype of older people always complaining about their aches and pains unfortunately is all too true. If you don't want to turn off your friends and family, complain to your doctor and no one else; or, better yet, follow this program so that you won't have any aches and pains—or at least, not as many.

It is also important to be aware of your interaction with others and the impact you are having on them. As you are talking, note their facial expressions and posture. If they are looking away, they probably are not giving you their total attention. It may be that you are prattling on and boring them, or it may be that something is distracting them. Check it out. Note their posture. Are their arms folded in front of them defiantly or hands on their hips in an "I dare you" stance? When they speak, are you truly listening to what they have to say? Most people are already planning and rehearsing their next response. Practice total listening as much as possible.

A GOOD NIGHT'S SLEEP

Have you ever heard the statement: "Oh, for a good night's sleep!"? The benefits of regular exercise program and a low-fat vegan diet are scientifically well founded. However, the benefits of sleep are often ignored. Poor sleep is a frequent complaint of seniors, and it seems to be more difficult to get a really good night's sleep as you age. Inadequate sleep can suppress your immune system; indeed, one sleepless night can lower the number of white blood cells in your body by twenty-eight percent.[3] Sleeplessness certainly affects energy levels and the ability to concentrate, and may even be associated with depression. During sleep is when the brain replenishes its supply of neurotransmitters such as dopamine. Recovery from the day's activities and healing from injury is accelerated during sleep.

There are two aspects of sleep that must be considered—the quantity and quality. Many people just don't allow enough time for sleep. Some regard sleeping as a waste of time and use drugs such as caffeine to stimulate their exhausted bodies into action. Some people allow plenty of time for sleep, but the quality of their sleep is poor. Vigorous, daily exercise is usually effective in helping people improve their ability to fall asleep. Physically fit people spend more of their sleeping time in deep sleep, and in REM (rapid eye movement) or dreaming sleep. These are the more restorative stages of sleep. People who are getting enough sleep wake spontaneously and feel refreshed.

According to research presented at the annual (2003) meeting of the American College of Sports Medicine, an increase in daily exercise can improve sleep quality among insomniacs.[4] Sleep researcher Shawn Youngstedt, PhD, suggests that if you have trouble sleeping, experiment with different intensities of exercise at different times of the day. If you find that you are having trouble getting to sleep, get up and do some quiet activity such as reading until you start to get drowsy. Also, get up at approximately the same time every morning, even if you have not had enough sleep, so that your body has a chance to maintain a regular schedule. Again, exercise will help even if you feel tired at first. Just keep going, and most of the time you will find yourself overcoming the lack of sleep and feeling back to normal. Then go to sleep at your usual bedtime.

MORNING AEROBIC EXERCISE HELPS SLEEP IN THE EVENING

Another study showed that women who exercised in the morning were able to sleep better at night.[5] In this research conducted at the Fred Hutchinson Cancer Research Center in Seattle, Washington, Shelley Tworoger, PhD, found that even stretching on a consistent basis improved sleep patterns. The yearlong study, which concluded in 2001, involved 173 women aged fifty to seventy-five who were overweight and did not take hormone replacement therapy. Before enrolling, all engaged in less than one hour of exercise each week and had trouble falling asleep without medication or staying asleep once they had fallen asleep.

The women were randomly assigned to an aerobic exercise or stretching program. Both groups had the option of working out in the morning or evening, and individuals sometimes chose to work out at home. The aerobic exercisers primarily walked or rode a stationary bike for forty-five minutes five times a week. Women who stretched attended sixty-minute stretching or relaxation sessions several times a week.

According to Dr. Tworoger, the results confirm the positive effect that regular morning exercise can have on sleeping patterns. Women who exercised in the mornings for a total of three to four hours a week had fewer problems falling asleep. Those who exercised for less than three hours a week did not experience this benefit. Women who exercised in the evenings had *more problems* falling asleep.

What accounts for the startling difference in morning versus evening exercise? Dr. Tworoger speculates that exercise may affect hormones that are involved in circadian rhythms (the body clock). Another possibility is that evening exercise raises the body temperature, which normally drops in preparation for sleep.

Stretching also has a positive impact on sleep—although not to the same extent as morning exercise—and it doesn't matter what time of day you do it. In the study, both women who stretched in the morning and those who stretched in the evening had less trouble falling asleep and used less sleep medication, says Dr. Tworoger.

So once again, getting your body moving—whether with aerobic exercise or simple, gentle stretches—turns out to be one of the vital keys to good health.

SLEEP-AID SUPPLEMENTS

We've discussed the risks of taking supplements in the chapter on diet. When it comes to sleep aids, many are enthusiastic about taking the popular sleep-aid supplement melatonin, a hormone produced by the pineal gland that governs our day/night cycles. A study done at Pennsylvania State College of Medicine suggests that melatonin may make symptoms worse for the half a million people who have a condition called orthostatic intolerance.[6] When they stand up, their bodies can't keep their blood pressure high enough to maintain blood flow to the brain, so they get dizzy and may faint. Normally, the body compensates by providing a change in blood pressure when standing up. Melatonin disrupts that mechanism. Sleeping pills are never the answer, either, because the body adapts to them and they are soon ineffective.

If you're still having trouble with getting good quality sleep, there are some basic principles of sleep hygiene to follow. For example, your sleep environment should include a bedroom that is darkened and quiet. This room should not be used for other activities such as watching television or study. The mattress should be the right degree of firmness, the bed sheets smooth, and the pillow should have the right degree of plumpness so that your head and neck are in proper alignment. Develop a pre-sleep evening routine of quiet activity, bathing, brushing teeth, journal writing, etc. Avoid stimulating activities such as television, arguing with anyone, and drinking any beverage with caffeine or alcohol. Try not to use an alarm to wake you up in the morning so that your body can determine when it's ready to awaken. Whether you awaken too early or too late, get up and go through your daily routine, and go to bed at your regular time. Most people find that taking naps interferes with a regular sleep routine, so avoid naps if that's the case with you. With a good diet and vigorous exercise program, you will have given your body its best chance at a good night's sleep.

Besides sleep, people often talk about having "a positive mental attitude" as important to good health and a long life. In my judgment, it is important to be realistic. Merely imposing a "positive" side on everything is a form of denial and is different from the reframing we talked about earlier. On the other hand, not being able to see the positives in every situation is also a form of denial. If you are eating a good diet and getting daily, vigorous exercise, your mental attitude reflects the state of health within. If you're not following the diet and exercising and feel terrible, your attitude is probably going to be negative no matter how hard you try to change it. In other words, a "positive mental attitude" can be the *result* of being fit, rather than the *cause*.

IMMUNIZATIONS

Although this can be a controversial subject, there is a great deal of evidence that some vaccines have very serious side effects, and some may not even be effective in the first place. The example of the 2003/2004 flu season is a case in point. The Centers for Disease Control and Prevention admits that the flu shot that was developed for that season was ineffective and that this has been the case for the past nine years. Vaccines sometimes also contain mercury as a preservative, and no one in their right mind would want mercury injected into their system. If you are following a low-fat, vegan diet and getting daily, vigorous exercise, your immune system should not be compromised and therefore should be able to handle any of the normal bugs that we are usually infected with.

SOME FINANCIAL IMPLICATIONS
FOR HEALTH CARE

There are so many good reasons to take care of our health and to be a fit senior. One that I have not mentioned much in this book is the financial one. If you take a look at the burgeoning costs of medical care—whether you are covered by Medicare, Medicaid, private insurance, or your own pocket—you will see an out-of-control financial disaster that is imminent. With our fiscal debt accumulating, some financial experts fear a total collapse of our economy. Former Secretary of the Treasury Robert Rubin states that we are "on an unsustainable path" and that "the scale of the nation's projected budgetary imbalance is now so large that the risk of severe adverse consequences must be taken very seriously."[7]

Besides the possible collapse of our economy, what good does a cure for cancer do us if it costs $50 million per person? According to the World Health Organization, the US is number one in the world in the incidence of degenerative diseases and twenty-sixth in life expectancy.[8] All of this is preventable, and very few politicians or private citizens are doing anything about it.

I hope that you will be in that category of those doing something about these problems. Some might ask, "What difference can just one person make?" Well, we all *already* make a difference—it's just that we choose whether the difference we make is *positive* or *negative*. Our choices in food and exercise make major differences to us, our economy, our environment, and the lives of the other creatures that inhabit this earth. We alone are responsible for the sad state of our health and others'. We are the ones who decide whether or not to frequent the fast food outlets, to buy foods soaked in pesticides, to put up with glitzy, excessive packaging, and to dump tons of our resources into the trash for someone else to take to the landfills. And it's only you and I that can stop this sick runaway train and start to reclaim our health and ensure that we have access to healthy, organic foods. If we don't support the people who produce organic fruits and vegetables, we will have no one to blame but ourselves when they are gone.

After my race this morning, one of my running/triathlete/senior buddies, Sharon Meindertsma, came up with an idea that she suggested I add to this book. She said, "You know how when you have an automobile accident, your car insurance rates go up? Well, our medical insurance premiums ought to go up if we don't follow the basic health-care guidelines such as keeping our weight, blood pressure and cholesterol within normal limits." She's suggesting that good health behavior should be rewarded financially with lower health insurance premiums, and, conversely, poor health behavior should be penalized to hit people in their pocketbooks just as poor driving does. It's an idea worth considering.

Of course, no matter how much you can afford to spend on health care, it's still better not to need it! Note that former President Bill Clinton, with access to the best medical care money can provide, still had to have heart bypass surgery to unblock clogged coronary arteries caused by eating the wrong foods.

HOW GOOD DO YOU WANT IT?

Today, life is so incredibly good that I sometimes have trouble comprehending all the changes in my life over the years since the cancer diagnosis. I've been sponsored by major corporations who have sent me all over the world to run races, and give talks and media interviews. I have a weekly radio show, "Nutrition & You," co-hosted by Terry Shintani, MD, and John Westerdahl, PhD, RD, and I get to talk to a variety of people who call in about their health concerns. I've been the keynote speaker at conventions and taught university-level courses such as "The Cancer Patient's Survival Guide" and "Focus on Health." I've given hundreds of talks to groups as diverse as elementary school kids, senior citizens groups, prostate cancer support groups, and medical conventions.

My first book, *A Race For Life*, was a way for me to encourage people to become "vegan triathletes." I'd gone from a totally sedentary "couch potato" to a casual mile-a-day plodder, to a world-class Ironman competitor. What I now know is that just about anybody can do it *if* they choose to. I also know that you don't have to go that far to get the benefits of boundless energy, that glow of radiant health on your face, a body that is lithe, sexy and lean, and delicious, wonderful sleep every night.

Just get up off that couch, put on some comfortable shoes, get yourself out of the door, and start out with a walk, if you have to. I started out running because it never occurred to me not to, and I was always in a hurry. Luckily, I was still young enough that there hadn't been too much damage to my body. However, you may have to walk in the beginning. As your body starts to respond, which it will immediately, you will soon find that you won't be able to help yourself as your body will just naturally want to break into a gentle jog, and then after a while, into a run. You'll feel the wind rustling through your hair, the spring in your step as you bound effortlessly up hills, and the thrill of transporting your body anywhere you want under its own steam.

I recall vividly the day I was competing in an ultra-marathon race up to the top of the extinct volcano Haleakala on the island of Maui. As I crossed the finish line, I looked back down at the thirty-seven miles I had just run and felt so proud of the legs that had taken me from sea level to 10,000 feet at the top. That accomplishment alone was exciting enough but to then be awarded a gold medal for first in my age group—wow, what a feeling!

Millions of people run every day, and it seems to me that the only ones who bad-mouth it are non-runners. I associate with the ones who run, love it, and who will tell you what a wonderful exercise it is. Last year I won two gold medals in our 2003 Senior Olympics, both in running events, and so did one of the listeners to our radio show. Sixty-three-year-old Beverly Page had heard me announcing the upcoming Senior Olympics, decided to show up, was the only one in her age group (60–64) and took home her first trophy. I think she's hooked! The real star of the show, however, was 101-year-old Erwin Jaskulski, who also took home the gold medal for running the 100 meters in 36:85!

In 2004, I reached thirty-six years of running. Running has been wonderful for my muscles, bones, joints, heart, lungs, tendons, ligaments, brain, and probably parts that I'm not even aware of. In fact, I can't think of any part of me that running has not been good for. Daily aerobic exercise of some sort—such as running, biking, swimming—is so important for everybody. If you put the right fuel in your tank (whole plant foods) and move it around faster by elevating the heart rate and literally adding more blood vessels, every cell in your body will thank you and sing the praises of this healthy lifestyle.

As a holder of world triathlon titles, I was still setting new records at the age of sixty-four. Kenneth Cooper, MD, president and founder of the world-famous Cooper Clinic in Dallas, Texas, the man who got me running in 1968 with his groundbreaking book *Aerobics*, follows my progress. According to his latest tests, he tells me there is no sign of cancer, and further, that this body of mine has exceeded the fitness level of "thirty-year-old superior category males."

This book has covered a fair amount of science and some of my own personal experiences. The purpose in this approach is twofold: Here is the theory that explains *why* these principles work; and here is the *application* of the theory to my own body and others, an answer to how I know what I know. While one can never generalize to a whole population, there is surely enough evidence—both from my own and others' experience and from studies—to draw the most basic of conclusions: that a vegan diet and vigorous exercise are worth a try.

Someone once said that "Education is not merely filling up the pail—it's lighting a fire." It's been the goal of this book to do both. The diet I espouse will prevent or reverse most diseases, and the exercise regimen I suggest will slow down the aging process and truly empower your "golden years."

You can't ask much more of a program than that!

Glossary

Amino acid: one of a group of twenty molecules making up the building blocks of protein

Arteriosclerosis: a thickening of the arteries with inflammatory changes

Atherosclerosis: arteriosclerosis with degenerative changes to the arteries

Bariatric: referring to the study of obesity

BMI: Body Mass Index, a calculated ratio of height and weight to determine obesity

Cataracts: a clouding of the lens of the eye

Cholesterol: a lipid molecule that is needed for making parts of the cell fabric as well as steroid hormones but leads, if deposited in artery walls, to atherosclerosis

Chromosome: a threadlike structure within the cell nucleus that carries the genes

Cohort studies: the use of similar or matched subjects in research studies

Corpus luteum: a structure formed from the follicle that after ovulation produces progesterone

Estrogen: the female sex hormone produced mainly but not exclusively in the ovaries

Follicle stimulating hormone (FSH): a pituitary hormone that causes ovarian follicles to grow and secrete estrogen

Follicle: a collection of cells within the ovary producing estrogen and containing a single egg cell

Free radical: an often highly reactive agent that can damage the cell and other molecules

Gene: the heritable unit of cells; there are about 70,000 different genes in human cells

Glaucoma: an increase in the pressure of the eye leading to damage of the optic nerve

Hormone replacement therapy (HRT): a chemical formulation of estrogen with or without progestin for treating symptoms of menopause

Hyponatremia: the condition of not enough electrolytes in the blood from drinking too much water

Infiltrating ductal carcinoma: a moderately fast-metastasizing form of breast cancer

Intraocular pressure (IOP): the pressure of the fluid in the eye that, if too high, leads to glaucoma

Macular degeneration: destruction of the macula, the part of the retina responsible for central vision

Melatonin: a hormone produced by the pineal gland during the hours of darkness that affects diurnal body rhythms

Menopause: the last menstrual cycle in a woman's life span

Monovision: the use of one eye for reading and the other for distance, achieved by either lenses or surgery

Orthostatic intolerance: a condition of inadequate blood to the brain upon standing upright

Osteoblasts: the cells in the bone that build new bone

Osteoclasts: the cells in the bone that break down old bone so it can be replaced by new bone

Osteoporosis: the loss of bone tissue and bony supports leading to fractures

Parenteral: feeding through the veins and not the intestinal tract

Pineal gland: a small gland attached to the brain that is responsible for secreting melatonin

Progesterone: a type of steroid hormone produced mainly by the ovaries and placenta that counterbalances estrogen

Progestin: the synthetic substitute for progesterone with many untoward side effects

Proprioceptors: the apparatus receiving stimuli caused by the actions of the body itself; muscle sense, which allows the body to maintain balance

Prostate gland: a gland at the base of the bladder in men that contributes to the formation of seminal fluid

Telomere: a cap on the end of chromosomes that does not contain a genetic code for proteins but has a protective function

Testosterone: the male sex hormone, mainly produced by the testes

References

INTRODUCTION

1. American Cancer Society. "Statistics." www.cancure.org/statistics.htm (viewed July 27 2004).
2. Cairns, John. "The treatment of diseases and the war against cancer." *Scientific American* 253:51 (November 1985).
3. McDougall, John MD. *The McDougall Program for Women: What Every Woman Needs to Know to Be Healthy for Life* (New York: Dutton, 1999).

CHAPTER 1—SENIOR FITNESS

1. Centers for Disease Control and Prevention. "Drug Deaths #4." *National Vital Statistics Reports, Deaths.* 49:8 (September 21 2001).
2. Menezes, Ravi J., et al. "Regular use of aspirin and pancreatic cancer risk." *Biomed Central Public Health* 2:18 (2002), www.biomedcentral.com/1471–2458/2/18 (viewed July 27 2004).
3. Blacklock, C.J., et al. "Salicylic acid in the serum of subjects not taking aspirin: comparison of salicylic acid concentrations in the serum of vegetarians, non-vegetarians, and patients taking low dose aspirin." *Journal of Clinical Pathology* 54(7): 553–555 (July 2001). Higher serum (blood) concentrations of salicylic acid were found in vegetarians (median 0.11 micromol/litre) than in non-vegetarians (0.07 micromol/litre). Although the median serum concentration of salicylic acid in patients taking aspirin (75 mg daily) was 10.03 micromol/litre, some of the vegetarians had higher levels than those taking the aspirin.
4. Costco Pharmacy, Honolulu, Hawaii, February 2004.
5. See www.cholesteroltest.org/chemicalcontrol.htm (viewed August 9 2004).
6. Vioxx was taken off the market by its manufacturer (not the FDA) years after the

FDA recognized an elevated risk of cardiac problems, 27,000 heart attacks and sudden cardiac deaths. "FDA Official Alleges Pressure to Suppress Vioxx Findings," Kaufman, Marc, *The Washington Post*, Oct. 6, 2004, www.washingtonpost.com

7. The statement refers to heartburn drugs in general and the study was reported in The *Journal of the American Medical Association*, Oct. 27, Laheij, Robert, University Medical Center, St. Radboud, Nijinegen, Netherlands.

8. "Hormone Replacement Therapy study stopped: overall health risks exceeded benefits." *Journal of the American Medical Association* 288(3): (July 17 2002).

CHAPTER 2—THE RIGHT DIET

1. Jacobson, Michael, quoted in *Nutrition Action Health Letter* (www.cspinet.org/nah), March 2004, "The government estimates that a lifestyle of poor diet and lack of exercise kills about 400,000 Americans every year—as many as smoking does."

2. Berenson, G.S., et al. "Atherosclerosis: a nutritional disease of childhood." *American Journal of Cardiology* 82(10B): 22T–29T (November 26 1998).

3. Bryant, William MD, and Dana Greer. "Plotting off the chart: obesity in children." www.pens.org/articles/greer-dana_obese1.htm (viewed July 27 2004).

4. Science NetLinks, a resource for science teachers (see www.sciencenetlinks.com). The estimate is approximately 10^{14} or 100 trillion cells, although the range is from 50 to 100 trillion.

5. Myant, N.B. *The Biology of Cholesterol and Related Steroids* (London: Heinemann Medical Books, Ltd., 1981), p. 611.

6. Sempos, C., et al. "The prevalence of high blood cholesterol levels among adults in the United States." *Journal of the American Medical Association* 262(1): 45–52 (July 7 1989). See also Sempos, C., et al. "Prevalence of high blood cholesterol among US adults: an update based on guidelines from the second report of the national cholesterol education program adult treatment panel." *Journal of the American Medical Association* 269(23): 3009–3014 (June 16 1993).

7. Campbell, T.C., et al. "Diet, lifestyle, and the etiology of coronary artery disease: the Cornell China Study." *American Journal of Cardiology* 26(82, 10B): 18T–21T (November 1998).

8. McMurray, M. "Changes in lipid and lipoprotein levels and body weight in the Tarahumara Indians after consumption of an affluent diet." *New England Journal of Medicine* 325(24): 1704–1708 (December 12 1991).

9. "Nutritionist III" computer program. Developed by N-Squared Computing of Salem, Oregon.

10. Slag, M. "Impotence in medical clinic outpatients." *Journal of the American Medical Association* 249(13): 1736–1740 (April 1 1983).

11. American Cancer Society. "Statistics." www.cancure.org/statistics.htm (viewed July 27 2004).

12. "Vegetables lower prostate cancer risk." *Journal of the National Cancer Institute* 92: 61–68 (January 5 2000).

13. Hill, P. "Environmental factors and breast and prostatic cancer." *Cancer Research* 41(9): 3817–3818 (September 1981).

CHAPTER 3—THE RIGHT EXERCISE

1. Cooper, Kenneth MD. *Aerobics* (New York: Bantam Books, 1968).

CHAPTER 4—AGING

1. Gosden, Roger. *Cheating Time: Science, Sex, and Aging* (New York: W.H. Freeman & Co., 1996).
2. Enos, W. "Pathogenesis of coronary disease in American soldiers killed in Korea." *Journal of the American Medical Association* 158: 912–914 (1955).
3. Ornish, Dean MD. "Intensive lifestyle changes for reversal of coronary heart disease." *Journal of the American Medical Association* 280(23): 2001–2007 (December 16 1998).
4. Esselstyn, Jr., Caldwell MD. "Updating a 12-year experience with arrest and reversal therapy for coronary heart disease." *American Journal of Cardiology* 84(3): 339–341, A8 (August 1 1999).
5. Carroll, K., "Experimental evidence of dietary factors and hormone-dependent cancers." *Cancer Research* 35(11 pt.2): 3374–3383, Review (November 1975).
6. World Health Organization. *World Health Statistics Annual* (Geneva 1989).
7. Smith, D.M. "The loss of bone mineral with aging and its relationship to hip fracture." *Journal of Clinical Investigation* 56: 311 (1975).
8 . Whalen, R. "Influence of physical activity on the regulation of bone density," *Journal of Biomechanics* 21: 825–837 (1988).
9. Blanchette, Patricia MD. Radio interview on "Nutrition and You." KWAI, Honolulu, Hawaii, 1998.
10. Wilmoth, J.R., et al. "Increase of maximum life-span in Sweden, 1861–1999." *Science* 289: 2366–2368 (September 29 2000). For other articles on increased life expectancy, see BBC News for May 9 2002 (http://news.bbc.co.uk/1/hi/health/1977733.stm) and Harry R. Moody, "Who's afraid of life extension?" (www.hrmoody.com/art5.html).
11. McDougall, John MD. *The McDougall Program* (New York: NAL Books/Dutton, 1990), pp. 85–86.
12. Fiatarone, Maria A., and W.J. Evans. "The etiology and reversibility of muscle dysfunction in the aged." *Journal of Gerontology* 48 Spec No: 77–83, Review (September 1993).

CHAPTER 5—WHY DIET MATTERS

1. Carpenter, K.J. "A short history of nutritional science: Part 2 (1885–1912)." *Journal of Nutrition* 133(4): 975–984 (April 2003).
2. www.glycemicindex.com (viewed July 28 2004).
3. Rose, W.C., and R.L. Wixom. "The amino acid requirements of man: XIII, The sparing effect of cysteine on methionine requirement." *Journal of Biological Chemistry* 216: 763–773 (1955).
4. Harris, W. *The Scientific Basis of Vegetarianism* (Honolulu: Hawaii Health Publishers, 1995), p. 154.

5. Lindler, M. *Nutritional Biochemistry and Metabolism* (New York: Elsevier Science Publishing Co. 1985), pp. 70–71.
6. Mensink, R.P., and M.B. Katan. "Effect of dietary trans fatty acids on high-density and low-density lipoprotein cholesterol levels in healthy subjects." *New England Journal of Medicine* 323(7): 439–445 (August 1990).
7. Picard, Andrew, et al. "Trans fats almost everywhere, tests find." *The Globe & Mail*, August 12 2003.
8. "Nutritionist III" computer program. Developed by N-Squared Computing of Salem, Oregon.
9. Quoted in Barnard, Neal MD. *The Power of Your Plate* (Summertown, Tennessee: Book Publishing Company, 1990), p. 15.
10. McDougall, John MD. *The McDougall Plan* (New York: New Century Publishers, 1983), pp. 41–42.
11. Burkitt, Denis. "Mean weight of stools and transit time in different populations." Cited in Keith Akers: *A Vegetarian Sourcebook* (New York: Putnam, 1983), p. 79.
12. Barnard, Neal MD. *Food for Life* (New York: Three Rivers Press, 1993), p. 71.
13. Campbell, T.C., et al. "Diet, lifestyle, and the etiology of coronary artery disease: The Cornell China Study." *American Journal of Cardiology* 26:82(10B): 18T–21T (November 1998).
14. Ibid.
15. DeRose, David J., et al. "Vegan diet-based lifestyle program rapidly lowers homocysteine levels." *Preventive Medicine* 30(3): 225–233 (March 2000).
16. Ridker, P.M., et al. "Comparison of C-reactive protein and low-density lipoprotein cholesterol in the prediction of first cardiovascular events." *New England Journal of Medicine* 347(20): 1557–1565 (November 14 2002).
17. Kendall, C., et al. "Effects of a dietary portfolio of cholesterol-lowering foods vs. lovastatin on serum lipids and C-reactive protein." *Journal of the American Medical Association* 290(4): 502–510 (July 23 2003).
18. Robbins, John. *The Food Revolution* (Berkeley: Conari Press, 2001).
19. "Lycopene: An Antioxidant for Good Health." See www.eatright.org/Public/ NutritionInformation/92_8300.cfm (viewed August 9, 2004).
20. Holt, Roberta R., et al. "Chocolate consumption and platelet function." *Journal of the American Medical Association* 287(17): 2212–2213 (May 1 2002).
21. Esselstyn, Jr., Caldwell MD. Television interview on "Tasty & Meatless," March 8, 2004.
22. Berney, D. "Vegetarian celebrities." *Vegetarian Times* 62 (1982), 70, and others.
23. "Physicians Committee for Responsible Medicine lawsuit versus the U.S. Department of Agriculture and the U.S. Department of Health and Human Services." See www.pcrm.org/news/lawsuit_summary.html (viewed July 28 2004).
24. Boileau, Thomas W.M., et al. "Prostate carcinogenesis in N-methyl-N-nitrosourea (NMU)-testosterone-treated rats fed tomato powder, lycopene, or energy-restricted diets." *Journal of the National Cancer Institute* 95(21): 1578–1586 (November 5 2003).
25. Fletcher, R.H., and K.M. Fairfield. "Vitamins for chronic disease prevention in adults: clinical applications." *Journal of the American Medical Association* 287(23): 3127–3129 (June 19 2002).
26. Heimendinger, J., and M.A. Van Duyn. "Dietary behavior change: The challenge of recasting the role of fruit and vegetables in the American diet." *American Journal of Clinical Nutrition* 61(6 Suppl): 1397S–1401S, Review (June 1995).

27. Watanabe, F., et al. "Pseudovitamin B-12 is the predominant cobalamide of an algal health food, spirulina tablets." *Journal of Agricultural and Food Chemistry* 47(11): 4736–4741 (November 1999).

28. Snow, C.F. "Laboratory diagnosis of vitamin B-12 and folate deficiency." *Archives of Internal Medicine* 159(12): 1289–1298 (June 28 1999).

29. McCaddon, A., et al. "Functional vitamin B-12 deficiency and Alzheimer disease." *Neurology* 58(9): 1395–1399 (May 2002).

30. Dhonukshe-Rutten, R.A., et al. "Vitamin B-12 status is associated with bone mineral content and bone mineral density in frail elderly women but not in men." *Journal of Nutrition* 133(3): 801–807 (March 2003).

31. DeRose, D.J., et al. "Vegan diet-based lifestyle program rapidly lowers homocysteine levels." *Preventive Medicine* 30(3): 225–233 (March 2000).

32. Wald, S., et al. "Homocysteine and cardiovascular disease evidence on causality from a meta-analysis." *British Medical Journal* 325(7374): 1202–1208 (23 November 2002).

33. Flicker, L., et al. "Serum vitamin D and falls in older women in residential care in Australia." *Journal of the American Geriatric Society* 54(11): 1533–1538 (November 2003).

34. Centers for Disease Control and Prevention. *National Vital Statistics Reports, Deaths: Final Data for 1999.* 49(8): 6 (September 21 2001).

35. Planin, E. "Cancer risk in farmed salmon." *The Honolulu Advertiser*, January 9 2004. Also featured in "What's wrong with fish?" *Vegetarian Times*, August 1995.

36. McMurray, M. "Changes in lipid and lipoprotein levels and body weight in the Tarahumara Indians after consumption of an affluent diet." *New England Journal of Medicine* 325(24): 1704–1708 (December 12 1991).

CHAPTER 6—EXERCISE—USE IT OR LOSE IT

1. Jakicic, J.M., et al. "Prescribing exercise in multiple short bouts vs. one continuous bout: effects on adherence, cardiorespiratory fitness, and weight loss in overweight women." *International Journal of Obesity Related Metabolic Disorders* 19(12): 893–901 (December 1995).

2. Cooper, K. MD. *Preventing Osteoporosis* (New York: Bantam, 1989), pp. 149–152.

3. Ibid., pp. 39–49.

4. Remy, Mark. "Calorie calculator." *Runner's World*, March 2004.

5. Lahr, D.D. "Does running exercise cause osteoarthritis?" *Maryland Medical Journal* 45(8): 641–644, Review (August 1996).

6. Fries, J.F., et al. "Running and the development of disability with age." *Annals of Internal Medicine* 121(7): 502–509 (October 1 1994).

7. Halpern, Brian MD, et al. *The Knee Crisis Handbook: Understanding Pain, Preventing Trauma, Recovering from Injury, & Building Healthy Knees for Life* (New York: Rodale Press, 2003).

8. Lane, N.E., et al. "The relationship of running to osteoarthritis of the knee and hip and bone mineral density of the lumbar spin: a 9-year longitudinal study." *Journal of Rheumatology* 25(2): 334–41 (February 1998).

9. Halpern, Brian MD, et al. See note 7.

10. Burke, Edmund, and Jay Kearney. *Optimal Muscle Recovery* (Vonore, Tennessee: Avery Publishing Group, 1999). (See www.optimalmusclerecovery.com.)

CHAPTER 7—REVERSING CARDIOVASCULAR DISEASE

1. Flapan, A.D. "Management of patients after their first myocardial infarction." *British Medical Journal* 309(6962): 1129–1134, Review (October 29, 1994).
2. Aronow, W.S., et al. "Prevalence of and association between silent myocardial ischemia and new coronary events in older men and women with and without cardiovascular disease." *Journal of the American Geriatric Society* 50(6): 1075–1078 (June 2002).
3. Castelli, W.P. "Cholesterol and lipids in the risk of coronary artery disease—The Framingham Heart Study." *Canadian Journal of Cardiology* 4Supp A: 5A–10A (July 1988).
4. Keys, A. *Seven Countries: A Multivariate Analysis of Death and Coronary Heart Disease* (Cambridge: Harvard University Press, 1980).
5. Jacques, P.F., Clarke, R. "Homocysteine and the risk of ischemic heart disease and stroke: a meta-analysis." *Journal of the American Medical Association* 288(16): 2015–2022 (October 23–30 2002).
6. For Greece, see: Trichopoulou, A., et al. "Adherence to a Mediterranean diet and survival in a Greek population." *New England Journal of Medicine* 348(26): 2599–2608 (June 26 2003). For Italy, Vannoni, F., et al. "Association between social class and food consumption in the Italian EPIC population." *Tumori* 89(6): 669-678 (November–December 2003). For Spain: Benach, J., et al. "The public health burden of material deprivation: excess mortality in leading causes of death in Spain." *Preventive Medicine* 36(3): 300–308 (March 2003).
7. Campbell, T. Colin, et al. "Diet, lifestyle, and the etiology of coronary artery disease: The Cornell China Study." *American Journal of Cardiology* 82(10B): 18T–21T (November 26 1998).
8. Ornish, Dean MD. "Intensive lifestyle changes for reversal of coronary heart disease." *Journal of the American Medical Association* 280(23): 2001–2007 (December 16 1998).
9. Esselstyn, Jr., Caldwell MD. "Updating a 12-year experience with arrest and reversal therapy for coronary heart disease." *American Journal of Cardiology* 84(3): 339–341, A8 (August 1 1999).
10. The 2002 VegSource conference. Dr. Esselstyn's words are online at vegsource.com/shopping/video_quotes.htm (viewed August 10, 2004).
11. Ibid.
12. Esselstyn, Jr., Caldwell MD. See note 9.
13. Bassler, Thomas MD. *The Whole Life Diet: An Integrated Program of Nutrition and Exercise for a Lifestyle of Total Health* (New York: M. Evans, 1979). "Marathoners are forever exempt from heart attacks," p. 10.
14. Plymire, D.C. "Running, heart disease, and the ironic death of Jim Fixx." *Research Quarterly for Exercise and Sport* 73(1): 38–46 (March 1 2002).
15. Harrison, P. "Walk-jog prescription introduced by Toronto centre now mainstay of cardiac rehabilitation." *Canadian Medical Association Journal* 149(4): 470–472 (August 15 1993).
16. Esselstyn, Jr., Caldwell, MD. See note 9.

CHAPTER 8—CANCER

1. National Cancer Institute, Bethesda, MD, cited in www.cancer2000.com/070199.html (viewed July 30 2004).
2. "Clinical implications of Surgeon General's Report on Smoking and Health." *Journal of the National Medical Association* 71(7): 713–715 (July 1979).
3. Centers for Disease Control and Prevention. *National Vital Statistics Reports, Deaths: 1987.*
4. Bommelaer, G., et al. "Epidemiology of intestinal functional disorders in an apparently healthy population." *Gastroenterology and Clinical Biology* 10(1): 7–12 (January 1986).
5. American Cancer Society, Screening Guideline, and Statistics, www.cancure.org/statistics.htm (viewed July 30 2004).
6. Vander Griend, D.J., and C.W. Rinker-Schaeffer. "A new look at an old problem: the survival and organ-specific growth of metastases." *Sci STKE* 2004(216): pe3–3 (January 13 2004).
7. Holm, L.E., et al. "Treatment failure and dietary habits in women with breast cancer." *Journal of the National Cancer Institute* Volume 85, Number 1 (January 6 1993).
8. Stripp, C., et al. "Fish intake is positively associated with breast cancer incidence rate." *Journal of Nutrition* 133(11): 3664–3669 (November 2003).
9. Mueller, C., et al. "Breast cancer in 3,558 women: age as a significant determinant in the rate of dying and causes of death." *Surgery* 83(2): 123–132 (February 1978).
10. McDougall, John MD. *McDougall's Medicine: A Challenging Second Opinion* (New York: New Century Publishers, 1985), pp. 30–34.
11. Campbell, T.C., et al. "Diet, lifestyle, and the etiology of coronary artery disease: The Cornell China Study." *American Journal of Cardiology* 26(82, 10B): 18T–21T (November 1998).
12. I quote from an email dated April 14 2004, written to me by T. Colin Campbell.
13. Carroll, K.K. "Experimental evidence of dietary factors and hormone-dependent cancers." *Cancer Research* 35: 3374–3383 (1975).
14. Ibid.
15. Lowenfels, A.B., et al. "Diet and cancer." *Cancer* 39(4 Suppl): 1809–1814 (April 1977).
16. Carroll, K.K. See note 13.
17. Wynder, E. "The dietary environment and cancer." *Journal of the American Dietetic Association* 71:385 (1977).
18. Eichner, Randy MD. "Physical activity as a modifiable risk factor." Physical Activity and Cardiovascular Health: National Institutes of Health, Consensus Development Conference Statement, December 18–20, 1995.
19. Burkitt, Denis. "Mean weight of stools and transit time in different populations." *Lancet* 2: 1408 (1972).
20. Blakely, L.J., et al. "Effects of pregnancy after treatment for breast carcinoma on survival and risk of recurrence." *Cancer* 100(3): 465–469 (February 1 2004).
21. Chang, K.J., et al. "Influences of percutaneous administration of estradiol and progesterone on human breast epithelial cell cycle in vivo." *Fertility and Sterility* 63(4): 785–791 (April 1995).
22. McGrath, Kris MD, cited in *Bottom Line/Health*, March 16, 2004.
23. Burkitt, Denis. See note 19.

CHAPTER 9—DIABETES

1. Gorman, C. "Why are so many of us getting diabetes?" *TIME* magazine, December 8, 2003, p. 60.
2. Ibid. p. 61.
3. Hogan, P., et al. "Economic costs of diabetes in the US in 2002." *Diabetes Care* 26(3): 917–932 (March 26 2000).
4. "Joint commission IDs five high-alert meds." *ED Management* 12(2): 21–22 (February 2000).

CHAPTER 10—OSTEOPOROSIS

1. Thomas, C.L., ed. *Taber's Cyclopedic Medical Dictionary* (Philadelphia: F.A. Davis Co., 1989).
2. Mazess, R., and W. Mather. "Bone mineral content of North Alaskan Eskimos." *American Journal of Clinical Nutrition* 27: 916–925 (September 1974).
3. Kanis, J., et al. "Calcium supplementation of the diet not justified by present evidence [Parts 1 and 2]." *British Medical Journal* 298: 137–149, 205–208 (1989).
4. Arnaud, C.D., and S.D. Sanchez. "The role of calcium in osteoporosis." *Annual Review of Nutrition* 10: 397–414 (1990). Also: "Symposium on human calcium requirements." *Journal of the American Medical Association* 185: 588–593 (1963).
5. Heaney, R.P., et al. "Calcium nutrition and bone health in the elderly." *American Journal of Clinical Nutrition* 36: 986–1013 (1982).
6. Cummings, S.R., et al. "Epidemiology of osteoporosis and osteoporotic fractures." *Epidemiology Review* 7: 178–208 (1985). Van Beresteijn, E.C., et al. "Relationship between the calcium-to-protein ratio in milk and the urinary calcium excretion in healthy adults." *American Journal of Clinical Nutrition* 52(1): 142–146 (1990). Abelow, B.J., et al. "Cross-cultural association between dietary animal protein and hip fracture: a hypothesis." *Calcified Tissue International* 50(1): 14–18 (January 1992). Some have claimed that Chinese women have high rates of osteoporosis, but Abelow shows that Chinese women have a low incidence of osteoporosis. Dr. Colin Campbell's findings support Abelow's research.
7. Walker, A.R., et al. "The influence of numerous pregnancies and lactations on bone dimensions in South African Bantu and Caucasian mothers." *Clinical Science* 42(2): 189–196 (February 1972).
8. Food and Agriculture Organization of the United Nations. *FAO Production Yearbook: 1986* (Rome, 1987).
9. US Department of Agriculture. "Nutritive value of foods." *Revised Home and Garden Bulletin* 72 (1981).
10. Heaney, R.P., and C.M. Weaver. "Calcium absorption from kale." *American Journal of Clinical Nutrition* 51(4): 656–657 (April 1990).
11. Beeson, P. L. *Cecil Textbook of Medicine* (Philadelphia: W.B. Saunders Co., 1979).
12. Margen, S., et al. "Studies in calcium metabolism: the calciuretic effect of dietary protein." *American Journal of Clinical Nutrition* 27: 584–589 (1974).
13. Zemal, M.B., et al. "Role of the sulfur-containing amino acids in protein-induced hypercalciuria in men." *Journal of Nutrition* 111: 545–552 (March 1981).
14. Personal email, dated April 15 2004.

15. Daniell, H. "Osteoporosis of the slender smoker. Vertebral compression fractures and loss of metacarpal cortex in relation to postmenopausal cigarette smoking and lack of obesity." *Archives of Internal Medicine* 136(3): 298–304 (March 1976).
16. Massey, L.K., et al. "The effect of dietary caffeine on urinary excretion of calcium, magnesium, sodium, and potassium inhealthy young females." *Nutrition Research* 4: 43–50 (1984).
17. Bockman, R. "Steroid-induced osteoporosis." *Orthopedic Clinics of North America* 21(1): 97–107 (January 1990).
18. Jones, H.H., et al. "Humeral hypertrophy in response to exercise." *Journal of Bone and Joint Surgery* 59A(2): 204–208 (March 1977).
19. Ibid.
20. Preliminary findings reported by the Osteoporosis Research Center from a researcher comparing bone density of walkers and runners.
21. Lindsay, R. "Bone response to termination of estrogen treatment." *Lancet* 1: 1325–1327 (1978).
22. Lee, J.R. *Natural Progesterone: The Multiple Roles of a Remarkable Hormone* (Sebastopol, California: BLL Publishing, 1994).
23. Ibid. See also Lee, J.R. *What Your Doctor May Not Tell You About Menopause* (New York: Warner Books, 1996).
24. Ibid. *Natural Progesterone.*
25. At the *os calcis* (heel), the average bone density is 411 mg/cm², which is measured by sending a small bit of radiation through the bone. The denser the bone, the less radiation passes through.
26. National Safety Council, *AARP* (*American Association of Retired People* magazine), July–August 2003, p. 6826. Martin, A.R., et al. "The impact of osteoporosis on quality of life: the OFELY cohort."
27. *Bone* 31(1): 32–36 (July 2002) and Fitzpatrick, P., et al. "Predictors of first hip fracture and mortality post fracture in older women." *Irish Journal Medical Science* 170(1): 49–53 (January–March 2001).
28. Sanson, Gill. *The Osteoporosis "Epidemic": Well Women and the Marketing of Fear* (New York: Penguin, 2001), pp. 25–29.
29. Pors Neilson, S. "The fallacy of BMD: a critical review of the diagnostic use of Dual X-ray Absorptiometry." *Clinical Rheumatology* 19(3): 174–183 (2000).
30. Freiherr, Greg. "Product promotion strategy links drugs and devices." *Medical Device & Diagnostic Industry* magazine, November 1995.

CHAPTER 11—ARTHRITIS

1. Fuhrman, Joel MD. "Autoimmune disease equals digestive dysfunction." *Fasting and Eating for Health* (New York: St. Martin's Press, 1998), pp. 146–149.
2. Atassi, M.Z. *Immunochemistry of Proteins* (Plenum Press 1977), p. 391.
3. Harris, William MD. *The Scientific Basis of Vegetarianism* (Honolulu: Hawaii Health Publishers, 1995), pp. 62–63.
4. Ibid. p. 63.
5. Atassi, M.Z. See note 2.
6. Khan, U., et al. "Modulation of the formation of adhesions during the healing of

injured tendons." *Journal of Bone Joint Surgery* (British Edition) 82(7): 1054–1058 (September 2000).

7. Panush, Richard MD. "Arthritis and exercise: alleged associations with osteoarthritis." Paper presented to American Medical Athletic Association, December 1998.
8. Van Aken, J., et al. "The Leiden Early Arthritis Clinic." *Clinical and Experimental Rheumatology* 21(5 Suppl): S100–S105, Review (September–October 2003).
9. McDougall J., et al. "Effects of a very low-fat diet in subjects with rheumatoid arthritis." *Journal of Alternative and Complementary Medicine* 8(1): 71–75 (February 2002).
10. Kauppila, L.I. "Can low-back pain be due to lumbar-artery disease?" *Lancet* 346(8979): 888–889 (September 30, 1995).
11. Ibid.
12. Tacconelli, S., et al. "Clinical pharmacology of novel selective Cox-2 inhibitors." *Current Pharmaceutical Design* 10(6): 589–601 (2004).

CHAPTER 12—HYPERTENSION AND DVTS

1. *Seventh Report of the Joint National Committee on Prevention, Detection, Evaluation, and Treatment of High Blood Pressure* (JNC 7).
2. McDougall, John MD. *The McDougall Program* (New York: NAL Books/Dutton, 1990), pp. 363–366.
3. Tudor-Locke, C., and D.R. Bassett, Jr. "How many steps/day are enough?" *Sports Med* 34(1): 1–8 (January 2004), and Ishikawa-Takata K., Ohta T., Tanaka H. "How much exercise is required to reduce blood pressure in essential hypertensives: a dose-response study?" *American Journal of Hypertension* 16(8): 629–633 (August 2003).
4. Cruickshank, J.M., et al. "Air travel and thrombotic episodes: the economy class syndrome." *Lancet* 2(8609): 497–498 (August 27 1988). Symington, I.S., Stack, B.H.R. "Pulmonary thromboembolism after travel." *British Journal of Diseases of the Chest* 71(2): 138–140 (1977).
5. Williams, A., et al. "Increased blood cell agglutination following ingestion of fat, a factor contributing to cardiac ischemia, coronary insufficiency and anginal pain." *Angiology* 8: 29–39 (1957).
6. Harris, William MD. *The Scientific Basis of Vegetarianism* (Honolulu: Hawaii Health Publishers, 1995), pp. 52–53.

CHAPTER 13—OBESITY

1. World Health Organization (2003). "Diet, nutrition and the prevention of chronic disease: 2003." WHO Technical Report Series 916, Section 5.2.
2. Gustafson D., et al. "An 18-year follow-up of overweight and risk of Alzheimer's disease." *Archives of Internal Medicine* 163(13): 1524–1528 (July 2003).
3. Centers for Disease Control and Prevention. *National Vital Statistics Reports, Deaths: Final Data for 1999.* 49(8): 6 (September 2001).
4. St-Onge, M.P., Heymsfield, S.B. "Overweight and obesity status are linked to lower life expectancy." *Nutrition Review* 61(9): 313–316, Review (September 2003). Khaodhiar, L., McCowen, K.C., Blackburn, G.L. "Obesity and its comorbid conditions." *Clinical Cornerstone* 2(3): 17–31, Review (1999).

5. Harris, William MD. *The Scientific Basis of Vegetarianism* (Honolulu: Hawaii Health Publishers, 1995), p. 60.

6. Gregg, E.W, et al. "Intentional weight loss and death in overweight and obese U.S. adults 35 years of age and older." *Annals of Internal Medicine* 138(5): 383–389 (March 4 2003).

CHAPTER 14—SEXY SENIORS

1. Lee, John MD. *What Your Doctor May Not Tell You About Menopause* (New York: Warner Books, 1996).

2. "NIH asks participants in women's health initiative, estrogen alone study to stop study pills, begin follow-up phase." National Institutes of Health Press Release, March 2, 2004. See www.nhlbi.nih.gov/new/press/04-03-02.htm (viewed July 30, 2004). Szabo, Liz. "Estrogen study may be ending." *USA Today*, March 1, 2004.

3. Liverman, C.T., and D.G. Blazer, eds. *Testosterone and Aging: Clinical Research Directions* (Committee on Assessing the Need for Clinical Trials of Testosterone Replacement Therapy, 2004).

4. New England Research Institute, *Conquering Erectile Dysfunction* video. See www.neri.org/html/products/product_details.asp?product_id=2 (viewed July 30, 2004).

5. Health Professionals Follow-up Study at the Harvard School of Public Health, www.hsph.harvard.edu/hpfs (viewed July 30, 2004).

6. Dorey, Grace, et al. "Pelvic floor exercises good for men, too." Study conducted at the Faculty of Health and Social Care at the University of West of England, Somerset Nuffield Hospital, Taunton, England.

7. Al Cooper. "Men's Orgasms Become Less Intense." Interviewed in *Bottom Line/Health*, June 1, 1998.

8. American Cancer Society. "Statistics." www.cancure.org/statistics.htm, viewed July 30, 2004.

9. Physicians Committee for Responsible Medicine. "Cancer Awareness Survey." *Good Medicine* 7 (Autumn 1999).

10. Reddy, B.S., et al. "Nutrition and its relationship to cancer." *Advances in Cancer Research* 32: 237–345 (1980).

11. "Premarin: Prescription for Animal Cruelty." Brochure produced by People for the Ethical Treatment of Animals. See www.menopauseonline.com/main.html (viewed July 30, 2004)

12. McPherson, K., and E. Hemminki. "Synthesizing licensing data to assess drug safety." *British Medical Journal* 328(7438): 518–520 (February 28, 2004). "HRT Risks 'Were Known Years Ago.'" BBC News story, February 27, 2004. See http://news.bbc.co.uk/2/hi/health/3492902.stm (viewed July 30, 2004).

13. Lee, John. See note 1.

14. Ibid.

15. "NIH asks participants. . . ." See note 2. Szabo, Liz. See note 2.

16. "HRT could affect ability to hear." BBC News story, February 25, 2004. See http://news.bbc.co.uk/1/hi/health/3516171.stm (viewed July 30, 2004).

17. "Study: HRT patients at higher risk for asthma" WBAL-TV, February 23, 2004. See www.thewbalchannel.com/health/2867850/detail.html (viewed July 30, 2004).

18. Pekhlivanov, B., et al. "Hysterectomy—a time for reappraisal." *Akush Ginekol* (Sofia) 38(1): 42–45 (1999).
19. http://www.urologychannel.com/bladdercontrol/index.shtml
20. Ibid.
21. McDougall, John MD. *The McDougall Program for Women* (New York: Dutton, 1999), p. 44.

CHAPTER 15—ALZHEIMER'S

1. Evans, D.A. MD, et al. "Alzheimer disease in the US population: prevalence estimates using the 2000 census." *Archives of Neurology* 60(8): 1119–1122. (August 18, 2003).
2. Regan, Michael. "Doctors debunk memory pills," Associated Press, *Honolulu Advertiser*, November 30, 2003.
3. Ibid.
4. Giem, P., et al. "The incidence of dementia and intake of animal products: preliminary findings from the Adventist Health Study." *Journal of Neuroepidemiology* 12(1): 28–36 (1993).
5. Mirkin, Gabe, MD. "Folic acid and Alzheimer's disease." (July 1, 2001), see www.drmirkin.com/nutrition/9218.html (viewed August 2, 2004).
6. DeRose, D.J., et al. "Vegan diet-based lifestyle program rapidly lowers homocysteine levels." *Preventive Medicine* 30(3): 225–233 (March 2000).
7. Alzheimer's Association estimate, Chicago, IL 2000. See www.alz.org.
8. Teri, L., et al. "Exercise plus behavioral management in patients with Alzheimer disease: a randomized controlled trial." *Journal of the American Medical Association* 290(15): 2015–2022 (October 15, 2003).
9. Gustafson, D., et al. "An 18-year follow-up of overweight and risk of Alzheimer disease." *Archives of Internal Medicine* 163(13): 1524–1528 (July 14, 2003).
10. Garza A.A., et al. "Exercise, antidepressant treatment, and BDNF mRNA expression in the aging brain." *Pharmacology, Biochemistry Behavior* 77(2): 209–220 (February 2004).
11. US Department of Agriculture. *Nutritive Value of American Foods Agricultural Handbook* (Washington, DC: Government Printing Office, 1975).
12. Manuelidis, E.E., et al. "Suggested links between different types of dementias: Creutzfeldt-Jakob disease, Alzheimer disease, and retroviral CNS infection, "*Alzheimer Disease and Associated Disorders* 3(1–2): 100–109 (Spring–Summer 1989).
13. Mulvihill, Keith. "Similarity seen in Alzheimer's and Mad Cow Disease protein," *Reuters Health Information*, August 26, 2000.
14. Manuelidis, E.E. See note 12.

CHAPTER 16—KEEPING YOUR SENSES

1. Couet, C., et al. "Lactose and cataracts in humans: a review." *Journal of American College of Nutrition* 10(1): 79–86 (February 1991).
2. Glaucoma Research Foundation. See http://www.glaucoma.org/treating/treatment/alt_meds.html.

3. Harris, William MD. "Is macular degeneration a dietary deficiency disease?" *The Island Vegetarian*, Vegetarian Society of Hawaii Newsletter (January–March, 2004).

4. Anderson, Robert MD, president and acting executive director of the American Board of Holistic Medicine, East Wenatchee, WA. Quoted in the *Holistic Studies Institute Newsletter*, December 2003.

5. McDougall, John MD. "Does aging cause hearing loss?" See www.hearinglossweb.com/Medical/Causes/aging.htm (viewed August 3, 2004).

6. Gosden, Roger. *Cheating Time: Science, Sex and Aging* (New York: W.H. Freeman, 1996), pp. 93–94.

7. Buchner, David MD. Interviewed in *Bottom Line/Health*, October 2003.

CHAPTER 18—PUTTING IT ALL TOGETHER

1. Blair, S.N., et al. "Physical fitness and all-cause mortality: a prospective study of healthy men and women." *Journal of the American Medical Association* 262(17): 2395–2401, (November 3, 1989).

2. Blair, S.N., et al. "Changes in physical fitness and all-cause mortality: a prospective study of healthy and unhealthy men." *Journal of the American Medical Association* 273(14): 1093–1098, (April 12, 1995).

3. Dept. of Psychiatry, Univ. of California, *Psychosomatic Medicine*, November–December, 1994, as cited in Cooper, Kenneth, *Can Stress Heal?* (Nashville, TN: Thomas Nelson Publishers, 1997), pp. 40–41.

4. Youngstedt, Shawn. Findings presented at the annual (2003) meeting of the American College of Sports Medicine. See www.acsm.org/publications/newsreleases2003/exercisesleep060603.htm (viewed August 3, 2004).

5. Tworoger, S., et al. "Effects of a yearlong moderate-intensity exercise and a stretching intervention on sleep quality in postmenopausal women." *Sleep* 26(7): 830–836 (November 1, 2003).

6. Rogers, N.L., et al. "Potential action of melatonin in insomnia." *Sleep* 26(8): 1958–1959 (December 15, 2003).

7. Quote from Robert Rubin, www.ustreas.gov/press/releases/rr3132.htm (viewed August 3, 2004).

8. World Health Organization, Statistics Information System, http://www3.who.int/whosis/hale/hale.cfm?path=whosis,burden_statistics,hale&language=english